UNFAIR CARE

Get the Healthcare You Deserve in a System Designed to Fail You

Dr. Bryan Laskin

Glowstick ™
P R E S S

230 Manitoba Ave South, Suite 110
Wayzata, MN 55391
bryanlaskin.com

Interior design and typesetting by Jess LaGreca, Mayfly book design

ISBN hardcover 978-1-7366437-7-8
ISBN paperback 978-1-7366437-8-5
ISBN ebook 978-1-7366437-9-2

Library of Congress Catalog Number: 2025912136
First printing: 2025

"*Unfair Care* is the missing map for those who feel frustrated, stuck, and lost in a healthcare system that wasn't designed to help them. But Dr. Bryan Laskin doesn't just diagnose the problems with the system, he hands you the tools to transform the care you receive. The current game may be rigged, but this book shows you how to stop playing by their rules and create your own game instead."

—Dan Sullivan, Co-Founder of Strategic Coach®

"Dr. Laskin shows how our broken healthcare system creates burdens for patients and clinicians alike. He understands that "can't get there from here" feeling that we doctors experience every day while battling to get our patients what they need. He outlines practical measures we can take right now, and creates a map for building a better system in the future."

—Dr. Allison Stolz, MD

"This book doesn't just expose and confirm what so many of us have long suspected; it proves that our healthcare system is rigged in favor of institutions and insurance companies that profit from withholding access to our own health data. Fortunately, Dr. Laskin doesn't stop at diagnosis. He offers the cure and a clear, actionable path for patients to take back control. A great read, and a powerful call to be part of the change."

—Paul Edwards, Founder of CEDR HR Solutions

"Raw. Honest. Transparent. Yet again, Bryan tackles difficult healthcare system truths head on—ones that aren't often voiced. More than ever patients are realizing they need to be in control of their health and care decisions. Access to your own health data is at a critical point as we see AI and personalized care transforming what providers can do. Thankfully Bryan does more than present the problem at hand, he artfully lays out the innovations, solutions and strategies needed to take healthcare into a bright future. I can't wait for changemakers to get their hands on this book!"

—Melissa Turner, BASDH, RDHEP, EFDA, Chief Hygiene Officer

"The system is stacked against you! Doctors, dentists and other healthcare professionals are good people, but they are practicing in a system that is designed by them, for them and to protect them. *Unfair Care* does a great job of unpacking the challenges the system creates for you as a patient. More importantly, it shares with you how to take back the control of your own care, and shows you the tools you can use to manage your own healthcare needs. A must read for anyone needing healthcare services—which is all of us!"

—Jason Woods, Healthcare Strategist

"*Unfair Care* is not a book any insurance company, hospital system, or even some health care providers want patients to have—but it's exactly the book every patient deserves. Dr. Bryan Laskin delivers a passionate, eye-opening exploration of the broken health care system, exposing the daily struggles patients endure, from fragmented information and systemic inefficiencies to profit-driven motives that put their well-being at risk. Through gripping stories and sharp analysis, the book critiques these flaws while offering hope and empowerment. Dr. Laskin provides a clear, actionable roadmap for individuals to take charge of their health, equipping them to confidently navigate daunting health care decisions. By cutting through the bureaucracy and urging patients to push past overburdened providers, restrictive insurance policies, and profit-hungry pharmaceutical companies, the book inspires a powerful shift, putting patients back in control of their health journeys. It's more than a critique—it's a rallying cry and a blueprint to reclaiming power in a flawed system."

—Dr. Maggie Augustyn, FAGD, FICOI, FAAIP,
practicing general dentist, author, inspirational speaker

"*Unfair Care* is fantastic. From the very first chapter, I was blown away by the powerful real-world stories. Dr. Laskin brings essential, practical knowledge to light in a way that is both deeply human and immediately actionable. I look forward to sharing this with others."

—Kathleen Adams, CFP® CPWA® RMA®
Founding Partner of Second 50 Financial

"Dr. Laskin nailed it with this book. *Unfair Care* is an excellent and insightful deep dive into the often frustrating and confusing world of modern-day western healthcare. Whether you are a healthcare provider or a patient, this book is essential to not only understanding the issues that affect us all, but what steps to take to start fixing the long-broken system."

—Dr. Brandon Tiek, DDS

"*Unfair Care* is a powerful and timely exploration of the vital connection between oral and overall health. With clarity and urgency, Dr. Bryan Laskin equips readers with practical tools to navigate the fragmented healthcare system and shows why truly integrated care is essential. This eye-opening book is a must-read for patients, health advocates, and providers alike."

—Jill Sirko, Ph.D.

"Prevention is where it all begins! As professionals we have the power to lead the way to truly help patients before they have chronic issues that we can help prevent. I say "knowledge is power" to my patients all the time, and the fast action tips and actionable items at the end of each chapter gives patients what they need to be their own advocates."

—Laura Bettencourt RDH and Hygiene Coach

Note to the Reader

The information presented in this book is intended for educational and informational purposes only. While every effort has been made to provide accurate, up-to-date, and reliable information, it is not intended to replace professional medical or legal advice, diagnosis, or treatment.

Not Medical Advice: The strategies, examples, and recommendations in this book should not be construed as medical advice. Your health situations and needs are unique. Always consult with qualified healthcare professionals before making significant changes to your healthcare approach, treatment plans, or medication regimens. The author and publisher are not responsible for any adverse effects resulting from the use of information contained in this book.

Not Legal Advice: Similarly, while this book discusses healthcare rights, insurance matters, and negotiation strategies, it does not constitute legal advice. Healthcare laws and regulations vary by state and change over time. Consult with a qualified attorney for specific legal questions related to your healthcare situation.

Global Relevance: While *Unfair Care* focuses primarily on navigating the United States of America healthcare environment, the vast majority of the concepts, strategies, and insights apply universally. Regardless of where you live, if you've ever felt like a bystander in your own health journey, this book is for you. Admittedly, some regulatory specifics or insurance practices may be U.S.-centric, but the underlying issues of data access, patient empowerment, and systemic inefficiency are global in nature. Wherever you are in the world, you'll find tools in these pages that can help you take control of your healthcare experience and demand better care.

Patient Stories: The patient stories and case examples throughout this book are either composite illustrations based on common healthcare experiences rather than accounts of specific individuals or real examples where the names have been changed. Names, personal details, and circumstances have been created to demonstrate concepts and strategies while maintaining privacy and confidentiality. Any resemblance to actual persons is coincidental.

Individual Results May Vary: The patient stories and examples described throughout this book represent specific individuals' experiences and outcomes. Your results may differ substantially based on your unique circumstances, health conditions, geographic location, insurance coverage, and the specific healthcare professionals and systems you encounter.

Research and Evidence Limitations: Healthcare research continually evolves. The information presented reflects understanding at the time of writing but may be subject to change as new evidence emerges. Always verify critical health information with current, authoritative sources.

Professional Relationships: While this book advocates for empowered partnership with healthcare professionals, it does not encourage confrontational or disruptive behaviors. Maintain respectful communication even when being assertive about your needs. The goal is productive collaboration, not antagonism.

Privacy and Security Considerations: When using any digital health platform, including apps for storing, sharing, or analyzing personal medical records, exercise extreme caution. Not all services are subject to HIPAA regulations. Always read privacy policies, avoid platforms that monetize user data, and choose tools that prioritize both encryption and transparent data use practices.

Financial Considerations: Cost estimates and financial strategies mentioned may not reflect current prices or be applicable in all regions. Always verify costs directly with clinics and insurance companies before proceeding with treatments or services.

Urgent Medical Needs: This book focuses on navigating routine and chronic healthcare situations. For medical emergencies or urgent health concerns, seek immediate professional medical attention by calling 911 or visiting your nearest emergency room. The strategies in this book are not designed for crisis situations requiring immediate intervention.

No Guarantees: Healthcare systems are complex and constantly changing. While the approaches described have helped many patients, the author and publisher cannot guarantee specific outcomes from implementing these strategies. Your experience will depend on many factors beyond the scope of this book.

By reading this book, you acknowledge these limitations and understand that you bear responsibility for your healthcare decisions. The author and publisher disclaim any liability for direct or indirect consequences that may result from using the information contained herein.

It is my sincere hope that this book empowers you to become an effective advocate for your healthcare while working collaboratively with qualified professionals who respect your partnership.

Better healthcare experiences are possible and you deserve nothing less.

To your health,
Dr. Bryan Laskin

Contents

Introduction: The Patient Revolution 1

Part I: Uncovering the Truth Behind Healthcare . . . 13

Chapter 1: Why the System Is Failing You 15

Chapter 2: Your Mouth as the Gateway to Your Health 33

Chapter 3: Dental vs Medical—What Each Gets Right

(and Wrong) 51

Part II: Taking Back Control 65

Chapter 4: Your Records, Your Rights 67

Chapter 5: Follow the Money 91

Chapter 6: How to Hack Better Care 115

Part III: Designing Your Care Model 129

Chapter 7: Build Your Personal Care Team 131

Chapter 8: Prevent First, Treat Smarter 151

Chapter 9: How to Demand More (and Get It) 169

Part IV: The Patient First Future 191

Chapter 10: Interoperability, AI, and the Rise of Smart Care . . 193

Chapter 11: From Passive Patient to Empowered Partner . . . 211

Conclusion: You're Not Waiting for the Future. You Create It. . . 219

References 225

Appendices & Extras 233

About the Author 275

Acknowledgements 277

INTRODUCTION

The Patient Revolution

"The secret of change is to focus all your energy not on fighting the old, but on building the new." —Socrates

"Everything looks normal. Your mammogram results are fine," Dr. Keller said with a reassuring smile, closing Ava's file with a gentle tap. "See you next year for your regular screening."

At fifty-one, Ava had been diligent about her annual mammograms, knowing that early detection was critical.

Three weeks later, however, Ava was working at her desk when she felt an unusual tingling sensation in her left breast. Not pain exactly, but something wasn't right. She tried to dismiss it, knowing her mammogram had been clear.

"It's probably nothing," she told herself. "The doctor said I was fine."

But standard mammography can miss up to 13% of breast cancers, especially in women with dense tissue (ACS 2022). This fact was not discussed during Ava's screening, despite her having dense tissue.

This critical information gap, between what patients know and what they need to know, is a recurring theme in healthcare today.

When the tingling persisted for a week, Ava's fear overpowered her initial denial, so she made an appointment with her primary care physician, who then referred her to a breast specialist. The specialist ordered an ultrasound followed by a biopsy of the suspicious area.

Ava received the phone call three days later, while sitting on her couch at home. "I'm sorry, Ava," the oncologist said, her voice solemn. "The biopsy results confirm that you have invasive ductal carcinoma. We need to schedule surgery as soon as possible."

The words hit like a physical blow. How could this happen when her mammogram had been clear just weeks ago? Ava felt betrayed by her doctors, and confused about what to do next.

Shockingly, false negatives in breast cancer screening happen more often than most patients realize, delaying diagnosis in approximately 10-30% of cases, with significant impacts on both treatment options and outcomes (Ciatto et al. 2007). For Ava, those statistics had become her reality.

"Will I need chemotherapy?" Ava's voice trembled as she asked.

"We'll know more after surgery," the oncologist explained. "The pathology report will tell us if the cancer has spread to your lymph nodes, which helps determine the stage and the appropriate treatment plan."

The lumpectomy was scheduled quickly. Ava spent the days before surgery in a fog of fear and disbelief, cycling through emotions. Shock that the cancer had been missed on her mammogram, anxiety about the surgery, and terror about what might come after.

Post-surgery, Ava woke to news that cut deeper than the surgical incisions.

"We found cancer in three of your lymph nodes," her surgeon explained. "This means the cancer is more advanced than we initially thought. Stage 3 rather than Stage 1."

The revelation was devastating. Ava was informed that her five-year survival rate dropped from the 99% for localized breast cancer to 86%, as the cancer had spread to regional lymph nodes (National Cancer Institute 2023).

These numbers that once seemed abstract in public health announcements now defined Ava's future. It was the first time her own mortality had been quantified so bluntly.

"Given the misdiagnosis from the initial screening and the lymph node involvement, I'd like to order a Cerianna PET scan," her oncologist suggested. "It's a newer molecular imaging test specifically designed for certain types of breast cancer. It could help us determine if there are estrogen receptors in other parts of your body that standard imaging might miss. This could significantly impact your treatment plan."

Ava nodded, determined to employ any option that could help ensure the most effective treatment. This specialized scan can change treatment plans in up to 16% of patients by detecting disease that standard imaging misses (Liu et al. 2019).

But two days later, on the Sunday before her test was scheduled, Ava received a call from the oncologist.

"I'm sorry, but your insurance has denied coverage for the Cerianna scan," the doctor said. "We've appealed, but they've denied it again."

When Ava asked why, she was told her case didn't meet the "medical necessity criteria" established by the insurance company. These criteria are often developed without considering anything regarding the individual patient's circumstances or the latest medical research.

Not wanting to wait the typical 3-4 weeks for another appeal process, as this is precious time when dealing with aggressive cancer, Ava asked about paying out-of-pocket.

"I don't have that information, but it costs thousands and thousands of dollars," the doctor replied vaguely. "We should cancel the test. Almost no patients pay for tests like this themselves. You can try calling the scheduler tomorrow, if you want."

Ava hung up the phone, tears of frustration streaming down her face. "Is this really an unnecessary test? It seems more like the insurance company trying to just save a buck," she thought.

The emotional toll of navigating a complex healthcare system while fighting for her life was overwhelming. Studies show that administrative barriers to care significantly increase psychological distress in cancer patients, with over a third, like Ava, reporting anxiety and depression specifically related to insurance and financial challenges (Zafar et al. 2013).

But Ava wasn't willing to give up. She contacted the hospital's financial services department directly and asked for the specific cost.

"I can't give price quotes over the phone, so we need to cancel the test," the financial coordinator said.

"Well then, I guess I will just show up and pay whatever it is," Ava replied.

"OK... the patient price is $3,200," the coordinator finally admitted.

"Three thousand?" Ava repeated. "But I was told it would cost 'thousands and thousands', implying it was so expensive no one could afford it!"

"Well, yes, the list price is higher, but the patient self-pay rate is $3,200."

Through her own research, Ava later learned that the hospital would have received approximately $8,000 from insurance had the test been approved, more than twice what she paid directly. This perverse financial structure meant the hospital had little motivation to help patients understand their actual out-of-pocket costs.

So, Ava kept her scheduled scan and paid the $3,200. While this is obviously a significant sum, it was one she could manage by withdrawing from her retirement savings.

The results proved critical. They revealed a small area of metastatic disease that had been missed on previous scans, fundamentally changing her treatment plan.

"Without this information, we would have under-dosed your therapy," her oncologist admitted. "And that could have cost you your life."

What troubled Ava most wasn't just the financial burden or the initial misdiagnosis. It was the realization that treatment decisions were being influenced by a financial structure that healthcare providers themselves likely did not fully understand.

For Ava and countless patients like her, navigating this system adds unnecessary emotional distress while forcing complex healthcare decisions to be made with incomplete information. Determined not to be a passive victim, Ava threw herself into learning everything she could about her health, fighting to take back control over her care.

As Ava told her support group: "Cancer tried to kill my body, but the healthcare system tried to kill my spirit."

The Brutal Truth

You are being misled.

As Ava's story teaches us, healthcare's complexity isn't an unfortunate accident. It's a business strategy. The convoluted maze of billing codes, insurance denials, prior authorizations, and network restrictions is intentionally designed to create friction and suppress utilization, all while maintaining the illusion of choice. These systems are not accidental inefficiencies. Rather, they are deliberate mechanisms put in place to elevate profitability by making care harder to access and understand (Cutler 2021).

I've witnessed this reality from multiple perspectives. As a practicing dentist for over two decades, I've seen how the system constrains even the most dedicated healthcare professionals. I've sat with patients confused by billing practices I couldn't fully explain. I've wrestled with insurance companies denying necessary care based on arbitrary guidelines. I've watched as artificial barriers between medical and dental care created dangerous gaps in patient treatment.

As a health technology entrepreneur, I've worked to create solutions that bridge the divisions separating different aspects of care. I've seen how resistant established systems can be to innovations that empower patients, even when those innovations could improve health outcomes and reduce costs.

And most personally, as a patient advocate, I've experienced the frustration of navigating fragmented care when my wife faced a serious health crisis made worse by poor information sharing between doctors. What started as a seemingly straightforward medical issue became a months-long odyssey through disconnected specialties, contradictory advice, and financial surprises. All while we were trying to focus on healing.

These experiences taught me that healthcare's problems aren't primarily about the people providing care. They are about the systems those people work within. Most healthcare professionals enter their fields with genuine passion to help others, only to find themselves trapped in structures that prioritize volume over quality, efficiency over connection, and billing over healing.

The evidence of this broken system surrounds us. Patients routinely encounter cryptic bills, hidden prices, and scattered medical records. For example, only about a quarter of hospitals fully comply with federal price transparency rules (PRA 2023). Meanwhile, insurance denials for necessary diagnostic services can delay critical treatment for weeks or months. This is time many patients simply don't have.

The consequences of this system extend far beyond financial burden. Patients must make life-altering decisions with incomplete information, coordinate their own care across disconnected clinicians, and advocate for themselves while battling illness. The emotional and physical toll is immense and largely unacknowledged by the system itself.

Consider how this plays out in everyday healthcare interactions. When you receive a bill weeks after treatment with charges you were never told about, it is likely not an oversight. It's a feature of a system designed to separate clinical care from financial reality. When your personal health records can't be easily transferred between clinicians, that's not a technical limitation. It's a strategy that creates dependence on those specific records systems. When prevention receives minimal emphasis compared to treatment, that's not ignorance about best practices. It's the result of financial incentives that reward intervention over wellness.

Yet there's another perspective worth considering: dedicated healthcare providers are equally frustrated, caught in the same dysfunctional system. Many physicians, nurses, dentists, and other professionals feel equally constrained by these structures that weren't designed to support healing relationships.

As one physician colleague confided to me: "I know spending more time with patients leads to better diagnoses and outcomes, but my schedule allows about 10 minutes per patient. I'm forced to interrupt patients within 30 seconds of them speaking. This isn't why I became a doctor."

Another doctor described the moral distress of knowing what care would best serve a patient but being unable to provide it due to insurance limitations or institutional policies. "I went into healthcare to help people, not to serve as a gatekeeper denying necessary care," she explained.

Nearly half of healthcare workers reported symptoms of burnout even before the pandemic, with many citing administrative burden and their inability to provide optimal care as primary factors (Office of the U.S. Surgeon General 2022).

The system isn't just failing patients. It's also failing the people trying to help them.

This mutual frustration creates a potential alliance between patients and doctors. When both sides recognize their shared interests in transforming healthcare delivery, meaningful change becomes possible. Many doctors welcome informed, engaged patients who understand the system's constraints and work collaboratively to navigate them.

Your Path to Empowerment

While the system has significant flaws, you have more power than you might realize. *Unfair Care* provides the guide for you to take command of your healthcare experience, regardless of how the system operates around you.

I've spent years developing, testing, and refining these approaches, first as a dentist seeking to provide truly patient-centered care, then as a healthcare entrepreneur creating tools to empower patients, and always as someone navigating the system for myself and my family. These aren't theoretical concepts, they're practical strategies that work within healthcare as it exists today.

In the pages that follow, you'll discover practical strategies to:

- **Access and control your complete healthcare information**, breaking down the artificial barriers between dental and medical records that compromise your care. You'll discover how to obtain, organize, and use your health data effectively. I'll show you exactly how to request records, what to do when you encounter resistance, and how to create a personal health information system that gives you the complete picture no single clinician typically has.

- **Decode the finances** driving healthcare decisions and use this knowledge to make more informed choices. You'll learn how to navigate insurance, understand pricing, negotiate costs, and avoid unnecessary expenses. We'll expose the hidden incentives shaping recommendations and how to separate financial considerations from clinical ones when evaluating options.

- **Build and manage your own healthcare team** that truly serves your needs. I'll show you how to select doctors, establish effective relationships, and coordinate care across specialties. You'll learn to identify practitioners who value partnership, techniques for facilitating communication between team members, and strategies for replacing doctors who don't meet your standards.

- **Transform from a passive recipient** of healthcare into an informed, empowered participant. You'll develop skills for productive appointments, shared decision-making, and effective self-advocacy. We'll cover how to prepare for visits, what questions to ask in different scenarios, and how to ensure your preferences are respected in treatment plans.

- **Leverage technology strategically** to create the connected care experience institutions have failed to deliver. From personal health records to remote monitoring tools, you'll learn which innovations genuinely enhance care and which primarily serve business interests. I'll guide you through evaluating digital health options and integrating them into your personal care strategy.

- **Navigate healthcare bureaucracy** with confidence rather than frustration. You'll master techniques for overcoming common barriers, resolving disputes, and ensuring your needs are met. We'll uncover insurance appeals, billing corrections, access challenges, and other administrative hurdles that often prevent patients from receiving optimal care.

Each chapter provides specific, actionable strategies illustrated through real patient experiences. You'll find scripts for difficult conversations, tools to organize your health information, frameworks for evaluating treatment options, and guidance for addressing common healthcare challenges.

These approaches have helped people like Ava take control of critical medical decisions. They've helped patients with chronic conditions receive more coordinated care across disconnected specialties. They've helped families avoid unnecessary procedures and unexpected costs. And they'll help you transform frustration and fear into confidence and clarity.

Importantly, you don't need to implement everything at once. Start with the strategies that address your most pressing healthcare challenges, then gradually incorporate others as you build confidence and experience. Even modest changes in how you approach healthcare can yield significant improvements in your experience and outcomes.

What This Book Is (and What it Isn't)

Unfair Care is not a guide to what you should eat, how to meditate, or which workout plan might change your life. It's not a wellness manual or another one-size-fits-all promise of better health.

There are already thousands of books offering advice in those areas, usually with more confidence than credibility. Some provide valuable insights. Many oversimplify complex health realities. Few address the fundamental challenge of navigating a healthcare system not designed with your best interests at the center.

This book focuses on something more fundamental: **giving you back command of your care**. It provides the understanding and tools to make smarter, safer, and more personalized decisions about your health.

Whether you're dealing with chronic illness, mental health challenges, or simply trying to avoid unnecessary procedures, real empowerment starts with **accessing and leveraging your health information**. That's where meaningful care begins, and that's where we'll focus our attention.

I created this guide after witnessing the artificial separation between patients and clinicians throughout my career, a division as problematic as the arbitrary split between oral and overall health. Both of these divisions persist for historical and financial reasons, not because they serve patients well.

My approach combines the clinical perspective I've gained as a healthcare provider with the patient perspective I've developed through personal and family experiences. This dual viewpoint allows me to translate between these worlds, helping you understand both the doctor's constraints and your own power within the system.

I won't pretend the strategies in this book will solve every healthcare challenge you face. Some system barriers remain stubbornly resistant to individual efforts. Some clinicians won't welcome your engagement. Some insurance policies will deny necessary care regardless of how skillfully you appeal.

But I can promise that implementing these approaches will significantly improve your healthcare experience. You'll face fewer surprises, make more informed decisions, receive more personalized care, and experience less discouragement navigating the system.

Most importantly, you'll transform from feeling helpless within a confusing system to feeling capable of directing your own care journey.

The Revolution Begins With You

Your health is too valuable to entrust to a system that consistently demonstrates its limitations. The time has come to reclaim control and actively reshape your care.

You are not helpless. You are not merely a passive patient at the mercy of impersonal institutions. You can become an informed participant who understands your rights, asks insightful questions, and actively contributes to your care.

Throughout this book, you'll gain the knowledge and tools to create meaningful relationships with your doctors, fostering mutual respect that significantly enhances your care. You'll learn to identify and work with healthcare professionals who value your participation rather than resist it.

This isn't merely theoretical. *Unfair Care* is a practical guide, including steps you can take right now. The healthcare system is complex, but your role within it doesn't have to be. You have the power to dramatically improve your care by becoming an effective advocate for your health.

The change you seek starts with understanding, grows through action, and thrives with persistence. You aren't waiting for the system to fix itself. You are becoming the catalyst for the healthcare you deserve.

Take command of your healthcare starting today. The first step is demanding full control over your health information. Not someday, but now.

This revolution starts with you.

PART I

Uncovering the Truth Behind Healthcare

ONE

Why the System Is Failing You

"Of all the forms of inequality, injustice in health is the most shocking and inhuman." —Dr. Martin Luther King Jr.

Imagine two people: James and Leah.

James visits his doctor for a persistent cough. After a brief 5 minute examination and a few standard questions, his doctor writes a prescription for an antibiotic and suggests he come back if symptoms persist. James leaves with medication but little understanding of his condition. But that is the doctor's job, anyway, right?

Two weeks later, his cough remains. A second opinion reveals he has mild asthma, a condition requiring entirely different treatment. Unfortunately, the unnecessary antibiotics disrupted his gut microbiome, causing digestive issues that would take months to resolve.

Leah experiences similar symptoms. Her doctor, however, spends twenty minutes discussing her medical history, lifestyle, and symptoms. Tests rule out common infections. Her doctor explains the diagnostic reasoning, suggests a pulmonary function test, and ultimately diagnoses adult-onset asthma.

Leah leaves with appropriate medication, a clear understanding of her condition, and a comprehensive management plan (without the months-long diarrhea that James endured).

Same symptoms. Same diagnosis. Two vastly different experiences. Two dramatically different outcomes.

This disparity isn't simply bad luck. The healthcare system James encountered was functioning exactly as designed, prioritizing volume and speed over thoroughness, prevention, and patient education.

Leah's experience demonstrates what's possible when the system serves the patient rather than itself. Unfortunately, this is an increasingly rare experience in American healthcare.

The Manufactured Complexity of Healthcare

Let's be clear: healthcare isn't inherently complex. It's been *made* complex.

Consider this scenario: you walk into a restaurant, order a meal, enjoy it, and pay the price listed on the menu. Simple, transparent, and predictable.

Now imagine walking into that same restaurant, ordering a meal without seeing a menu, eating whatever they bring you, and then receiving a bill thirty days later.

But the bill doesn't come from the restaurant. It comes from separate entities representing the chef, the server, the ingredients, the table, the chair, and the building. Each charges different amounts using codes you don't understand for services described in language that seems deliberately obtuse.

Would you eat there again? Of course not. Yet this is precisely how healthcare operates.

This complexity serves specific purposes: it conceals true costs, creates dependency on intermediaries, shifts power away from patients, and obscures accountability. When you can't easily compare prices or understand what you're paying for, clinicians and insurers can maintain inflated costs without accountability. When you can't understand the system, you become passive, accepting whatever care (and costs) you're given rather than demanding what you actually need.

When you need an MRI, your doctor refers you to a particular imaging center (often without discussing alternatives), your insurance may require pre-authorization (a process that can take weeks), and you likely won't know the actual cost until after the procedure. What's hidden is that MRI prices can vary by 500% or more within the same geographic area for identical services. A knee MRI might cost $425 at one facility and $2,500 at another, with no difference in quality.

💡 Fast Action Tip

Always ask before any procedure:

"Can you provide a cost estimate and tell me if it needs prior authorization?"

This single question can save you thousands of dollars and months of frustration.

These complications are not just annoying, they directly affect care quality. Studies confirm that increased administrative burden and convoluted systems are linked to delayed diagnoses, decreased patient satisfaction, and even higher mortality rates (Sinsky et al. 2016; Makary and Daniel 2016).

Also, this complexity disproportionately harms those with limited time, education, or language proficiency. Those with fewer resources face nearly insurmountable barriers when trying to advocate for themselves.

The Information Asymmetry Problem

Healthcare's power hierarchy begins with information. Specifically, who has it and who doesn't.

Consider Mike, a waiter who experienced chronic fatigue for years. Despite multiple doctor visits, lab tests, and medications, his condition persisted.

Frustrated, he finally requested his complete medical records. After studying them, he noticed his thyroid levels had been consistently at the very edge of the "normal" range. Though not technically abnormal, Mike wondered if these borderline levels were significant given his symptoms.

He researched thyroid function and found studies suggesting some patients experience symptoms despite test results within standard ranges. At his next appointment, he discussed these findings with a new endocrinologist who agreed to try a low-dose thyroid medication. Within weeks, Mike's energy returned. He had lost years of his life to fatigue not because treatment was impossible, but because he lacked access to his own information.

This knowledge gap is no accident. Healthcare systems historically controlled patient data, releasing it reluctantly and often incompletely. Even now, and despite federal regulations supporting patients' right to their records, many clinics make accessing your information difficult through fees, delays, and bureaucratic hurdles.

Why? Because information is power. When you can't see your complete records, test results, or treatment options, you remain dependent on clinicians to interpret that information for you. This dependency maintains traditional healthcare power dynamics, where doctors dictate and patients comply.

Moreover, healthcare data remains frustratingly divided. Your primary care physician may not have access to your dental records, despite growing evidence linking oral health to systemic conditions. Your specialist might never see test results ordered by another doctor, leading to redundant procedures and uncoordinated care. This division dangerously contributes to misdiagnoses, drug interactions, and treatment delays.

The solution seems obvious: give patients control of their complete health information. But this simple fix threatens the status quo, where gatekeeping information maintains professional authority and financial advantage.

The communication problem extends to the language used in healthcare itself. Medical terminology often serves as a barrier rather than a bridge to understanding. When a physician tells you that you have "idiopathic peripheral neuropathy" rather than "nerve pain with no clear cause," they reinforce their position as the exclusive interpreter of your condition.

True informed consent requires understanding both the benefits and risks of all available options, including the option to do nothing. Yet many patients often receive incomplete information that emphasizes benefits while minimizing risks.

The consequences of this knowledge imbalance are particularly severe for marginalized communities. Research consistently shows that Black patients receive less information about treatment options and less time for questions during clinical encounters than White patients with identical conditions (IOM 2003). This information disparity directly contributes to healthcare inequities and poorer outcomes among minority populations.

EMPOWERED PATIENT PYRAMID

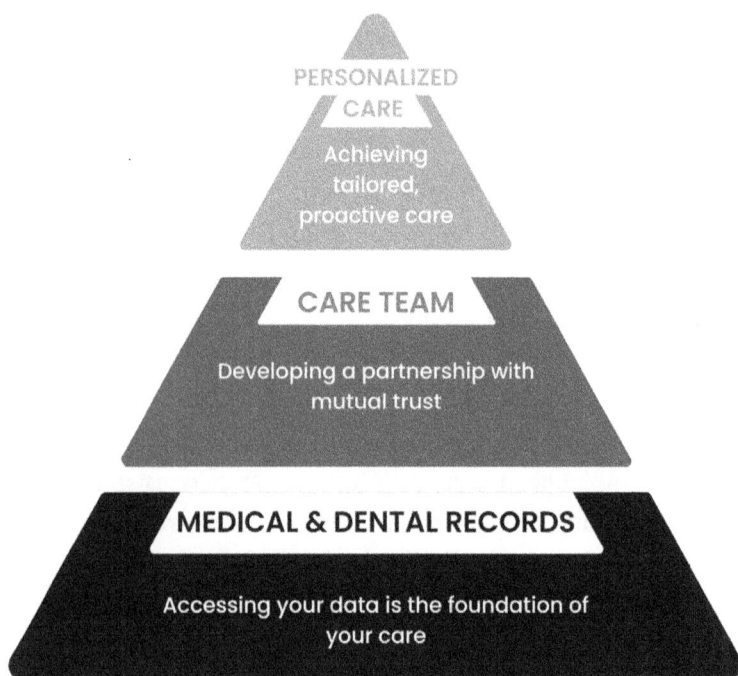

PERSONALIZED CARE
Achieving tailored, proactive care

CARE TEAM
Developing a partnership with mutual trust

MEDICAL & DENTAL RECORDS
Accessing your data is the foundation of your care

The Prevention Paradox

Our healthcare system excels at crisis intervention but fails miserably at prevention.

According to the CDC, 90% of the nation's $4.1 trillion in annual healthcare expenditures goes toward treating chronic and mental health conditions, many of which are preventable (CDC 2024). Meanwhile, less than 3% of healthcare spending goes toward prevention (CMS 2023).

This imbalance isn't accidental. Our system rewards dramatic interventions, such as emergency surgeries, intensive drug regimens, and heroic end-of-life measures, while offering minimal compensation for prevention. A hospital receives tens of thousands of dollars for treating a heart attack but pennies for helping patients prevent one.

A dental practice earns significantly more from an extraction and implant placement than from teaching effective oral hygiene that might have saved the tooth.

Consider Ellen's story. At 52, she was diagnosed with advanced periodontal disease requiring extensive treatment. Looking back at her dental records, she discovered that early signs had been present for years; slight bleeding noted during check-ups and some gum recession mentioned in passing. But her dentist had never emphasized the seriousness of these symptoms or explained how they might progress. The system largely ignores prevention and rewards procedures instead.

Ellen eventually lost three teeth and faced over $12,000 in treatment costs, potentially preventable with early intervention and education. Even more concerning, periodontal disease is linked to increased risk of cardiovascular conditions, potentially affecting her overall health.

This neglect of prevention extends to our entire healthcare infrastructure. We build massive hospitals for treating disease but invest comparatively little in community wellness centers. We spend billions on medications for chronic conditions but relatively little on nutrition education, stress reduction programs, or accessible exercise facilities that might prevent these conditions in the first place.

It has been proven that countries that prioritize preventive care consistently achieve better health outcomes at lower costs. The Netherlands, for example, spends significantly less per capita on healthcare than the United States while achieving better outcomes across numerous metrics (Schneider et al. 2021). The key difference? Their system financially incentivizes preventive care and early intervention rather than expensive treatments for advanced disease.

The prevention gap is particularly notable in dental care. Studies repeatedly demonstrate that every dollar invested in preventive dental care saves between $8 and $50 in restorative treatments, yet our insurance structures and practice models continue to undervalue prevention (Nasseh et al. 2017). Many dental insurance plans cover only the most basic preventive services while imposing significant cost-sharing for even minor restorative procedures. This creates financial barriers that discourage patients from seeking the very care that would save them money and discomfort in the long term.

Perhaps most disheartening is how the prevention paradox affects children. Early childhood interventions, from prenatal care to developmental screening to dental sealants, all yield enormous long-term health benefits and cost savings. Yet these services remain chronically underfunded and inconsistently provided, setting up future generations for preventable health problems that will require expensive interventions later in life.

The Fragmentation Failure

Perhaps nothing better illustrates healthcare's dysfunction than its persistent disconnection between different aspects of care.

Jennifer learned this lesson the hard way. Diagnosed with rheumatoid arthritis, she diligently followed her rheumatologist's treatment plan, including powerful immunosuppressant medications. During this time, she developed a tooth infection but didn't mention her arthritis medication to her dentist, unaware of its relevance. Her dentist, without access to her complete medical record, prescribed an antibiotic that interacted poorly with her immunosuppressant, leading to a severe reaction that required hospitalization.

The dangerous disconnect between medical and dental care is endemic to our system. Oral health directly impacts overall health, from heart disease to diabetes to pregnancy outcomes, yet dental care remains separated from medical care in both practice and insurance coverage. This artificial division reflects historical developments and professional boundaries rather than sound healthcare delivery.

This division extends beyond the medical-dental divide. Specialists rarely communicate effectively with primary care providers. Mental health remains separated from physical health. Alternative therapies exist in parallel universes from conventional medicine. And electronic health record systems, supposedly designed to facilitate information sharing, often can't communicate with one another.

When healthcare professionals operate in isolation, they develop tunnel vision, focusing exclusively on their specialized domain while missing crucial connections to overall wellbeing. The cardiologist treats the heart without considering the mouth; the dentist treats the teeth without considering the heart. The patient, whose body functions as an integrated system, suffers from this disjointed approach.

The problem becomes even more acute for patients with multiple chronic conditions. These patients often see five or more specialists, each managing a separate condition with minimal coordination. The result is polypharmacy (multiple medications prescribed by different doctors), contradictory advice, and treatment plans that may work at cross-purposes.

Consider Robert, a 68-year-old with diabetes, hypertension, and arthritis. His endocrinologist prescribed a medication that raised his blood pressure, complicating his hypertension management. His cardiologist, unaware of his worsening arthritis pain, recommended an exercise regimen that his rheumatologist would have considered inappropriate. His dentist, unaware of his cardiac condition, didn't provide appropriate antibiotic prophylaxis before a dental procedure, putting him at risk for endocarditis. Each doctor was competent within their specialty, but without coordination, their combined care was potentially harmful.

Electronic health records (EHR) were supposed to solve this problem, but in many ways, they've made it worse. Most EHR systems were designed primarily for billing rather than clinical care coordination, and different healthcare systems use incompatible platforms. The result is a digital divide that mirrors and reinforces professional silos.

Even within the same healthcare system, separation of data persists in subtle ways. Mental health records may be separated from physical health records due to privacy concerns. Imaging results might be stored in systems separate from clinical notes. Laboratory values may be difficult to track over time. This technical disconnection makes it nearly impossible for clinicians, let alone patients, to see the complete picture of a person's health.

✋ **Pause and Remember**

Your body is one system. Your health data should be too.

When information is scattered, mistakes multiply. When it's unified, healing accelerates.

The costs of these divisions are enormous. Duplicate testing, conflicting treatments, preventable hospitalizations, and medical errors all stem directly from our inability to coordinate care effectively. It is estimated that this disconnection costs the U.S. healthcare system approximately $765 billion annually, about 25% of total healthcare spending (IOM 2013).

The Patient as Product

Perhaps most fundamentally, today's healthcare system fails because it no longer sees patients as partners, but as products.

In the early days of medicine, healthcare was relationship-based. doctors knew their patients personally and understood their lives and values. Treatment decisions emerged from dialogue and shared decision-making. This approach didn't ensure perfect outcomes, but it did ensure that care aligned with what mattered most to patients.

Today's industrialized healthcare has largely abandoned this model. Driven by metrics, protocols, and profit margins, modern healthcare processes patients through streamlined pathways with minimal attention to individual circumstances. The eight-minute appointment, the checkbox-driven electronic health record, the assembly-line surgery center, all reflect a system designed for throughput rather than healing.

This transformation of care turns patients from people into revenue sources. Your value to the system isn't measured by your health outcomes but by the procedures you receive, the medications you take, and the billable encounters you generate. Your time, comfort, dignity, and preferences become secondary considerations.

The consequences extend well beyond dissatisfaction. When patients feel processed rather than heard, they become disengaged from their own care. They withhold crucial information, fail to follow treatment recommendations, and avoid seeking care until conditions become severe. This disengagement leads to poorer outcomes and higher costs, a lose-lose situation for everyone except those profiting from the revolving door of chronic illness.

Hospital room layouts prioritize clinician convenience over patient comfort. Appointment scheduling systems maximize provider productivity rather than patient access. Even the language reflects this shift. Patients have become "consumers," care has become "service delivery," and healing has become "clinical outcomes management."

This mindset pervades medical education as well. New physicians are trained to diagnose and treat disease efficiently but receive minimal training in communication, empathy, or shared decision-making. The implicit message is that technical competence matters more than human connection.

The system measures success through metrics like wait times, procedure volumes, and revenue per encounter. Rarely does it measure whether patients feel heard, understood, or empowered.

When patients express concerns about their care, they're often channeled through customer service protocols designed to placate rather than address root causes. Complaints become "customer service opportunities" rather than signals of systemic problems requiring meaningful change.

This transactional approach creates particular harm for those already marginalized by society. When healthcare becomes a transaction rather than a relationship, those with the least social capital, often racial minorities, non-English speakers, elderly patients, and those with disabilities, experience the greatest disadvantages. Their unique needs and circumstances become inconvenient variations in standardized processes rather than essential considerations in personalized care.

Dr. Karen's Transformation

Dr. Karen's story illustrates both the system's failures and the possibility of something better.

For fifteen years, Dr. Karen practiced internal medicine in a large healthcare system, seeing thirty patients daily in rushed appointments. She excelled at diagnosis and treatment but increasingly felt she was shortchanging her patients. "I was practicing what I call 'halfway medicine,' identifying problems but never having time to fully address them or prevent them from recurring," she recalls.

The breaking point came when her own father received a delayed cancer diagnosis despite multiple visits to his primary care physician. "He kept having the same symptoms, but in those short appointments, there was never time to connect the dots," Dr. Karen explains. "By the time they figured it out, his options were limited."

Determined to practice differently, Dr. Karen made a radical change. She opened a direct primary care practice where she would see no more than twelve patients daily and spend at least thirty minutes with each. She eliminated insurance bureaucracy, instead charging a transparent monthly membership fee that covered unlimited visits, virtual consultations, and basic procedures.

The results were transformative for both Dr. Karen and her patients. Freed from volume-based incentives and administrative burdens, she could focus on thorough evaluation, education, and prevention. Her patients received not just treatment but understanding of their conditions and partnership in their care.

"One of my patients had been to five specialists for chronic fatigue," Dr. Karen recalls. "In our first, full-hour appointment, I reviewed her complete history and noticed patterns suggesting a rare autoimmune condition that had been missed. We confirmed it with testing and started appropriate treatment. She later told me that having a doctor who had time to listen literally gave her life back."

Dr. Karen's practice isn't just more satisfying, it's more effective. Her patients experience fewer hospitalizations, require fewer specialist referrals, and report higher satisfaction than comparison groups in traditional practices. "When you remove the unreasonable pace and artificial time constraints," she notes, "good medicine becomes possible again."

This model represents a fundamental shift from reactive to proactive, from myopic to holistic, from doctor-centered to patient-centered care. Most importantly, it restores the essential relationship between patient and doctor that drives meaningful healthcare.

What makes Dr. Karen's story particularly compelling is that her transformation didn't demand extraordinary resources or specialized training. It only required the courage to practice medicine aligned with her values rather than system demands. Her success demonstrates that many of healthcare's failures stem not from inherent limitations but from artificial constraints that could be removed with sufficient will.

The direct primary care model Dr. Karen adopted isn't the only alternative to traditional fee-for-service medicine. Across the country, innovative clinicians are experimenting with approaches that realign incentives, restore relationships, and improve outcomes. These alternatives share common elements: They prioritize time for meaningful interaction, emphasize prevention, reduce administrative burden, and measure success by patient outcomes rather than procedure volumes.

Dr. Karen's experience highlights another crucial reality: healthcare clinicians themselves are often as frustrated with the current system as patients are. Many entered their profession with the genuine intent to focus on healing people, but find themselves trapped in structures that prevent them from practicing according to their values. When given the opportunity to practice differently, many embrace alternatives that better serve both patients and their own professional fulfillment.

This mutual dissatisfaction creates potential for alliance and change. When patients and doctors recognize their shared interest in transforming healthcare, they become powerful advocates for systemic reform rather than adversaries in a dysfunctional system.

Taking Control: Your Path Forward

The healthcare system's failures are systemic, but your response doesn't have to be passive acceptance. Throughout this book, you'll discover practical strategies to navigate, challenge, and ultimately transform your healthcare experience. But meaningful change begins with three fundamental principles:

1. **Claim ownership of your health information.** Your medical and dental records belong to you, not to the systems that created them. Access to your complete health data is not a privilege but a right, one increasingly supported by federal regulations like the 21st Century Cures Act. By gathering and controlling your health information, you gain the foundation for informed decision-making.

2. **Seek transparency in all healthcare interactions.** Demand clear explanations of diagnoses, treatment options, and costs before making decisions. Question recommendations that seem rushed or one-size-fits-all. Remember that genuine healthcare partners welcome informed questions rather than discouraging them.

3. **Build your own integrated care team.** Don't wait for our archaic healthcare systems to communicate to each other. Become the connector that ensures your doctors share crucial information. Seek out practitioners who value collaboration and patient partnership, even if that means changing providers.

These principles aren't just philosophical. They're practical steps toward healthcare that actually serves your needs. The chapters ahead will equip you with specific tools, scripts, and strategies to implement them effectively.

The path to better healthcare isn't about finding perfect doctors or perfect systems. Such perfection doesn't exist. Rather, it's about becoming an active participant in your care. It's about recognizing that while you didn't create healthcare's systemic problems, you have significant power to mitigate their impact on your personal health.

This journey begins with understanding the forces that shape your healthcare experiences. But knowledge alone isn't enough. In the chapters that follow, you'll learn specific, actionable techniques for applying this understanding to create immediate improvements in your care.

You'll discover how to:

- Evaluate doctors based on their willingness to partner with you
- Prepare for appointments to maximize their effectiveness
- Appeal insurance denials successfully
- Research treatment options independently
- Coordinate care across multiple clinicians
- Build relationships with your doctors that foster mutual respect

These skills don't require medical training or specialized knowledge, just clarity about your rights, confidence in your ability to act, and commitment to your wellbeing. By developing these capabilities, you transform from a passive recipient of care to an active participant in your health.

Action Items

Knowledge without action creates awareness but not change. As you process the realities described in this chapter, consider taking two immediate steps:

1. **Request your complete medical records** from all your healthcare providers. Under federal law, you have the right to these records in electronic format. While some clinicians may create bureaucratic hurdles, persistence pays off.

These records are the foundation for becoming an informed healthcare participant.

2. **Download the Cair app** to begin taking control of your dental records. This mobile application allows you to access, organize, and share your dental information, eliminating one critical information gap in your healthcare.

You can download the Cair app at cair.net, or just scan the QR code below:

Note: I Co-Founded Cair because I believed that no adequate tools existed for patients. It's one option, but not the only one. Choose the tools that work best for you.

For guidance on requesting your records effectively, including template letters and scripts for overcoming common obstacles, visit **unfaircare.com/resources**. There, you'll find additional tools specifically designed to help you implement the principles discussed in this chapter.

The healthcare system may be failing you, but have the power to change your healthcare experience. By understanding the structural problems behind your frustrating experiences, you've taken a large step toward something better. The power to change your healthcare experience begins not with policy reforms or system overhauls, but with your decision to no longer accept the unacceptable.

Your healthcare transformation starts now. Not next year. Not after the next policy change.

The system is counting on your continued passive acceptance. Prove it wrong.

TWO

Your Mouth as the Gateway to Your Health

"The mouth is the mirror of general health and disease, the sentinel of disease, and the gateway to your body."
—Sir William Osler

When Angela, a 45-year-old mother of four, visited her dentist for a routine cleaning, she expected the usual polite reminder about flossing more regularly. Instead, her dentist noticed something concerning; her gums showed signs of significant inflammation despite her diligent home care routine. The dentist also observed unusual white patches on the sides of her tongue.

Rather than simply scheduling a deep cleaning, her dentist asked about recent health changes. Angela mentioned fatigue, unexplained weight loss, and frequent minor infections. She had dismissed these symptoms as work stress.

Her dentist suggested she get tested for immune system concerns. The nonjudgmental tone, compassion, and professionalism with which he approached the conversation gave Angela the courage to follow through with testing, despite her initially finding it an odd suggestion, coming from her dentist.

The result was devastating; HIV infection. Angela was overwhelmed with shock, fear, and a flood of questions about her future and her family. "I remember sitting in my car after getting the results, unable to drive home, just sobbing," she recalled. "Everything I thought I knew about my life suddenly seemed uncertain."

However, the comprehensive support she received ended up positively transforming Angela's experience. Her dentist immediately connected her with a support group specifically for women with HIV. "He didn't just identify a health issue and send me on my way," Angela explained. "He recognized the emotional earthquake this diagnosis would cause and made sure I had both medical and emotional support from day one."

With proper medical treatment initiated early, Angela's viral load was quickly suppressed to undetectable levels. Perhaps as importantly, the psychological support helped her work through the complex emotions and adjust to her new reality. "Without the counseling and peer support, I might have spiraled into depression," she acknowledged.

Two years later, Angela remains deeply grateful to her dentist who saw beyond her teeth to her overall health. "The oral symptoms in my mouth weren't just dental issues, they were my body's early warning system," she reflected. "My dentist's willingness to look at me as a whole person literally saved my life. And not just medically, but by connecting me with the emotional support I needed to face this diagnosis with courage, rather than despair."

Angela now shares this message with others, stating, "A doctor who treats you as a complete person rather than a set of symptoms can make all the difference. Not just in clinical outcomes, but in how you experience the road from illness to wellness."

Angela's story illustrates a basic truth that our disconnected healthcare system often ignores: your mouth isn't isolated from the rest of your body. It's intricately connected to your overall health, functioning as both indicator and influencer of your wellbeing. The artificial separation between dental and medical care doesn't just create inconvenience. This separation is dangerous, obscuring crucial connections that could lead to better prevention, earlier diagnosis, and more effective treatment.

The Mouth-Body Connection: Not Just Teeth

One of the most damaging fractures in our broken healthcare system lies hidden in plain sight, the artificial separation between dentistry and medicine.

The relationship between oral health and systemic health works in both directions. Your mouth affects your body, and your body affects your mouth. This isn't alternative medicine or fringe theory, it's established science supported by decades of research.

Consider these documented connections:

- **Heart Disease**: People with gum disease are 2-3 times more likely to have a heart attack, stroke, or other serious cardiovascular event (Tonetti and Van Dyke 2013). The inflammation-causing bacteria in your mouth don't stay there. They travel through your bloodstream, potentially triggering inflammation in your arteries. This is so significant that some cardiologists now recommend periodontal evaluation as part of a cardiac risk assessment.

- **Diabetes**: This relationship works both ways. Diabetes increases your risk of developing gum disease, while untreated gum disease makes blood sugar control more difficult. Treating gum disease can improve diabetes management as effectively as some medications. Studies show that periodontal treatment can reduce HbA1c levels (a measure of long-term blood sugar control) by approximately the same amount as adding a second diabetes medication (Simpson et al. 2010).

- **Pregnancy Complications**: Pregnant women with gum disease face significantly higher risks of preterm birth and low birth weight (Offenbacher et al. 1996). These complications can have lifelong consequences for children.

The inflammatory substances released from infected gums can enter the bloodstream and potentially affect the development of the fetus and the stability of the pregnancy. Some studies suggest that periodontal treatment during pregnancy may reduce these risks (Michalowicz et al. 2006).

- **Respiratory Conditions**: Bacteria from gum disease can be inhaled into the lungs, potentially causing or worsening pneumonia and chronic obstructive pulmonary disease (COPD) (Sjögren et al. 2008). For elderly or immunocompromised patients, this mouth-lung connection can be particularly dangerous. Improving oral hygiene in nursing home residents may lead to significantly reduced pneumonia rates (Zimmerman et al. 2020).

- **Rheumatoid Arthritis**: Research has identified links between the bacteria associated with gum disease and rheumatoid arthritis. Some studies suggest that treating gum disease may reduce arthritis symptoms (Hashimoto et al. 2015). The inflammatory processes in the mouth may trigger or exacerbate the inflammatory processes in the joints, creating a vicious cycle of chronic inflammation.

- **Cognitive Function**: Emerging research indicates associations between poor oral health and cognitive decline, including Alzheimer's disease (Dominy et al. 2019). While the exact mechanisms continue to be studied, inflammation appears to play a key role. Oral bacteria and their byproducts have been identified in brain tissue from Alzheimer's patients, suggesting a potential direct link between oral pathogens and neurodegenerative changes.

These connections aren't merely statistical associations. They reflect biological processes through which oral health directly impacts overall health. Gum disease creates a chronic inflammatory state, releasing inflammatory substances that travel throughout the body. Oral bacteria enter the bloodstream through inflamed gum tissue, potentially affecting distant sites. The immune response to oral pathogens may trigger autoimmune reactions affecting other organs.

> ### Did You Know?
>
> Treating gum disease can lower your blood sugar as much as adding a second diabetes medication, without the side effects.

Yet our healthcare system continues to treat the mouth as if it exists in isolation from the rest of the body. This is clinically harmful, hiding crucial early warning signs and preventing integrated approaches to chronic disease management.

Consider David, a 58-year-old with well-controlled type 2 diabetes who suddenly developed persistent high blood sugar despite no changes to his medication, diet, or exercise. After months of confusion and increasing medication doses, his endocrinologist finally asked about his oral health. A dental examination revealed significant gum infection. Once treated, David's blood sugar levels rapidly improved, allowing him to reduce his medication. Those months of poor glucose control could have been avoided had dental and medical care been connected from the start.

Or take Maria, age 62, who saw multiple specialists for persistent, unexplained fatigue. She underwent extensive testing, including blood work, cardiac evaluation, and sleep studies. All showed minimal abnormalities. No one asked about her oral health until she mentioned jaw pain to her primary care physician. A dental evaluation revealed extensive infection in a tooth with a previous root-canal that showed no obvious symptoms other than mild discomfort. Within weeks of treatment, Maria's energy returned. The body-wide inflammation caused by her dental infection had manifested primarily as systemic fatigue rather than localized pain.

These cases aren't anomalies, they are examples of a pervasive problem created by our siloed approach to healthcare. What makes this particularly unfortunate is that the mouth provides uniquely accessible diagnostic opportunities. Unlike most organs, which require invasive procedures or advanced imaging to examine, the mouth can be directly visualized and monitored with minimal intervention. This accessibility makes oral health indicators potentially valuable for early disease detection, but only if we connect both dental and medical perspectives.

The Invisibility of Dental Disease

Part of what makes the mouth-body connection easy to overlook is the often silent progression of dental disease. Unlike many medical conditions that announce themselves with pain or visible symptoms, oral health problems frequently develop invisibly until they become quite advanced.

Early gum disease rarely causes pain. Cavities often remain symptom-free until they reach the nerve. Even oral cancers frequently progress silently, detected only when they become particularly advanced. This silent progression allows conditions to worsen before treatment, often necessitating more invasive, expensive interventions than would have been required with earlier detection.

When an early-stage dental infection doesn't cause obvious mouth pain, patients and doctors rarely connect it to seemingly unrelated symptoms like fatigue, mild cognitive changes, or increased blood sugar.

The problem is compounded by widespread dental anxiety. Approximately 36% of Americans experience dental fear, with 12% suffering from extreme dental anxiety (Beaton et al. 2014). This fear leads many to avoid regular dental visits, creating a dangerous cycle: avoidance leads to worsening conditions, which eventually require more invasive treatments, reinforcing anxiety and further avoidance.

THE CYCLE OF AVOIDANCE

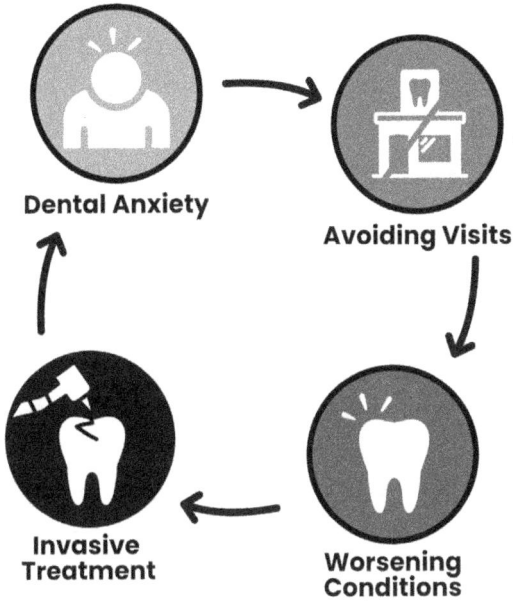

Dental Anxiety

Avoiding Visits

Invasive Treatment

Worsening Conditions

Even for those without dental anxiety, our healthcare system creates structural barriers to connected care. As dental and medical records exist in separate systems, neither dentists nor physicians have complete information. When dental and medical insurance operate independently, with different coverage, networks, and payment models, patients face a fractured system that makes coordinated care almost impossible.

The consequences extend beyond individual patients to population health. Dental disease remains one of the most prevalent yet preventable health conditions in America. More than 90% of adults have experienced dental cavities, while nearly half of all adults over 30 show signs of gum disease (CDC 2019). These aren't simply cosmetic concerns. They are infections with whole-body implications, potential signposts to systemic disease, and sources of chronic inflammation that can worsen numerous health conditions.

Inflammation: The Common Denominator

To understand how your mouth affects your overall health, we need to understand inflammation, as it is the common denominator connecting these seemingly disparate systems.

Inflammation is like a slow-burning fire in your body. In the short term, it's protective, helping eliminate infections, clear damaged tissue, and initiate healing. But when inflammation becomes chronic, persisting for months or years rather than days, it transforms from protective to destructive, potentially damaging healthy tissues and organs throughout your body.

Gum disease represents a textbook example of chronic inflammation. The bacterial biofilm that initiates gum disease triggers an inflammatory response that, without intervention, becomes self-perpetuating. The resulting chronic inflammation doesn't just damage gum tissue and bone. It releases inflammatory substances into the bloodstream, potentially triggering or worsening inflammation elsewhere in the body.

This oral-systemic inflammatory connection helps explain many of the associations between gum disease and systemic conditions. Heart disease, diabetes, rheumatoid arthritis, and Alzheimer's all involve inflammatory components. When gum disease adds additional inflammatory burden, these conditions often worsen. Conversely, reducing oral inflammation through gum treatment can sometimes improve management of these systemic conditions.

Take, for example, Gregory, a 67-year-old with rheumatoid arthritis who experienced increasingly severe flares despite aggressive medication. His rheumatologist suggested a comprehensive dental evaluation, which revealed moderate gum disease that Gregory hadn't noticed, as it caused no pain and minimal bleeding. After treatment, his arthritis symptoms improved significantly, allowing his rheumatologist to reduce his medication dosage.

Gregory's case illustrates how addressing inflammation in your mouth can provide a missing piece in managing systemic inflammatory conditions. His story isn't unique. Research increasingly suggests that dental treatment may complement medical management for various inflammatory diseases (Hajishengallis 2015).

Yet our healthcare system rarely connects these approaches. Physicians rarely consider oral health status when managing inflammatory conditions. Dentists typically lack access to patients' complete health records, limiting their ability to identify potential systemic implications of their findings. And insurance structures discourage interconnected care, with dental treatment almost never being covered by medical insurance, even when it might improve medical outcomes and reduce the cost of care.

The Bacterial Highway

Beyond inflammation, oral health impacts systemic health through direct bacterial transmission. Your mouth harbors over 700 species of bacteria. Some of these species are beneficial, some harmful, most context-dependent. However, it is particularly true that when gum disease or dental decay occurs, harmful bacteria can multiply, creating ideal conditions for infection. Also, gum disease creates pockets between teeth and gums, where these bacteria gain direct access to your bloodstream.

This "bacterial highway" can allow harmful bacteria from your mouth to travel to distant parts of your body, potentially contributing to infections elsewhere. Oral bacteria have been identified in heart valves, brain tissue, and joint fluid. While their presence doesn't prove causation, mounting evidence suggests these bacteria may directly contribute to disease processes beyond the mouth.

The bacterial connection appears particularly significant for cardiovascular disease. Multiple studies have identified oral bacteria in arterial plaque, suggesting these organisms may contribute directly to plaque formation or destabilization. Some of these bacteria can cause blood platelets to clump together, potentially increasing clotting risk. Others produce enzymes that may damage arterial walls, promoting atherosclerosis.

For patients with certain heart conditions, this bacterial highway creates specific risks. Individuals with artificial heart valves, previous endocarditis, certain congenital heart defects, and cardiac transplants face increased risk of infective endocarditis, a potentially life-threatening infection of the heart's inner lining or valves. For these patients, even routine dental procedures can allow oral bacteria to enter the bloodstream and potentially colonize vulnerable cardiac tissue.

This risk is well-established enough that clinical guidelines recommend preventive antibiotics before dental procedures for high-risk cardiac patients. Yet many patients aren't aware of these guidelines or don't understand which cardiac conditions qualify as high-risk. Meanwhile, communication gaps between cardiologists and dentists mean that cardiac patients often receive either inadequate protection or unnecessary antibiotics, both resulting in problematic outcomes.

The bacterial highway doesn't just affect the heart. Pneumonia, particularly in hospitalized or institutionalized patients, often involves inhalation of oral bacteria into the lungs.

Oral Hygiene Saves Lives

Studies in nursing homes have shown that improving dental hygiene can significantly reduce pneumonia rates among residents, a vivid demonstration of how oral bacteria can directly fuel deadly respiratory infections. (Sjögren et al., 2008)

Even brain health may be affected by oral bacteria. Research has identified bacteria associated with gum disease in brain tissue from Alzheimer's patients (Dominy et al. 2019). These bacteria produce substances that have been linked to neural damage characteristic of Alzheimer's disease. While this research remains preliminary, it suggests potentially direct mechanisms connecting oral bacteria to neurodegenerative disease.

Despite these bacterial connections, our healthcare system rarely addresses the mouth as a potential source of systemic infection. Patients hospitalized for serious infections seldom receive oral health evaluations as part of their workup. Those with recurrent infections rarely have their oral health assessed as a potential contributing factor. And preventive strategies that might reduce bacterial transmission from your mouth to the rest of your body receive minimal attention in most medical settings.

Beyond Gum Disease: Other Oral-Systemic Connections

While gum disease receives the most attention in discussions of oral-systemic health, other dental conditions also impact overall wellbeing.

Sleep apnea, a disorder characterized by repeated breathing interruptions during sleep, often has oral origins or manifestations. Dentists may identify anatomical risk factors like narrow airways, enlarged tonsils, or retracted jaws during routine examinations. They can also recognize signs of teeth grinding that frequently accompany sleep apnea. For many patients, dental appliances offer effective first-line treatment for mild to moderate sleep apnea, potentially reducing cardiovascular risks, improving energy, and enhancing quality of life.

Temporomandibular disorders (TMD) affect approximately 10 million Americans, causing jaw pain, headaches, ear pain, and facial discomfort. Beyond their direct symptoms, these disorders can impact nutrition (when pain limits chewing), sleep quality, and mental health

(NIH 2023). The intimate connection between jaw muscles, facial nerves, and the cervical spine means that TMD can both cause and result from problems elsewhere in the body.

Oral cancer kills approximately 11,000 Americans annually, more than cervical cancer, Hodgkin's lymphoma, or testicular cancer (ACS 2023). Early detection dramatically improves survival rates, and dental professionals are ideally positioned to identify suspicious lesions before they become symptomatic. Yet oral cancer screening remains inconsistent, and public awareness of oral cancer risk factors and warning signs remains low.

Eating disorders often manifest first with oral symptoms, as frequent vomiting (in bulimia) or nutritional deficiencies (in anorexia) damage teeth and oral tissues. Dentists may notice signs like enamel erosion, enlarged salivary glands, or lesions on the palate before patients display obvious weight changes or admit to disordered eating. This early detection opportunity can facilitate intervention before significant medical complications develop.

Autoimmune conditions like Sjögren's syndrome, lichen planus, and pemphigus often present with oral manifestations before affecting other parts of the body. Dentists who recognize these conditions can facilitate early diagnosis and treatment, potentially preventing serious complications.

These connections underscore the mouth's role as both sentinel and gateway for overall health. A visible, accessible site where systemic conditions often show early signs, and where prompt intervention might prevent progression.

Yet our healthcare system rarely capitalizes on these opportunities, treating oral findings as isolated dental concerns rather than potential indicators of broader health issues.

The Economic Consequences of Disconnection

Beyond its clinical impact, the separation between dental and medical care creates significant economic inefficiencies for individual patients, insurers, and the broader healthcare system.

For individual patients, the economic consequences manifest in multiple ways. Preventable emergency department visits for dental conditions cost patients and insurers approximately $1.7 billion annually, expenses that could be avoided with routine dental care (Wall and Vujicic 2015). Patients with chronic conditions like diabetes and heart disease spend an estimated 40% more on medical care when they have untreated gum disease, costs that might be reduced with connected care approaches (Jeffcoat et al. 2014).

For insurers, the division creates counterproductive economic incentives. Medical insurers have little motivation to cover dental treatments that might reduce medical costs, since those savings might accrue to a different dental insurer. Dental insurers, meanwhile, have little financial benefit to emphasize the systemic health implications of oral conditions, as doing so might suggest they should cover more preventive and therapeutic services.

For our overall healthcare system, these misaligned priorities translate into significant, yet preventable, spending. One report estimated that better integration of dental and medical care could save the U.S. healthcare system up to $100 million annually through reduced hospitalizations, emergency visits, and chronic disease complications (Nasseh et al. 2014).

The economic case for care coordination becomes particularly compelling when considering specific conditions. For pregnant women, comprehensive gum care costs far less than the neonatal intensive care required for premature infants. Yet many insurance plans don't cover gum disease treatment during pregnancy.

For diabetic patients, the cost of regular dental care pales in comparison to the expense of managing diabetes complications that might be worsened by gum inflammation. Unfortunately, however, medical necessity coverage for dental care remains rare for diabetic patients.

These economic realities create a troubling dynamic where short-term cost avoidance drives decisions that ultimately increase everyone's long-term expenses. A classic example of how our siloed system prioritizes immediate financial concerns over both patient wellbeing and long-term economic sustainability.

Reclaiming Connected Health: Your Action Plan

Despite these structural problems, you can take specific steps to bridge the dental-medical divide and ensure your oral health contributes positively to your overall wellbeing:

1. **Communicate comprehensively with all clinicians.** Ensure your dentist knows your complete medical history, including all medications and chronic conditions. Similarly, make sure your physician knows about any dental conditions, treatments, or concerns. Don't assume this information is shared automatically. It rarely is.

2. **Request coordinated care when appropriate.** If you have a condition with known oral-systemic connections (like diabetes, heart disease, or pregnancy), ask both your physician and dentist how they might coordinate your care. Remember, specific questions prompt specific answers; vague concerns generate vague responses.

3. **Document and share your own records.** Since healthcare systems rarely share information effectively, become the connection point. Request copies of both dental and medical records, and bring relevant information to all appointments. Digital tools, like the Cair app, can help organize this information for easy sharing.

4. **Understand your risk factors and warning signs**. Educate yourself about how your specific health conditions might affect or be affected by your dental health. This knowledge helps you recognize potential concerns before they become serious problems.

5. **Advocate for appropriate preventive care**. If you have a condition that increases your dental risk (like diabetes or certain medications), discuss with both your dentist and physician what preventive strategies might help. This might include more frequent dental visits, specialized home care products, or modified treatment approaches.

These strategies won't fix the structural problems in our healthcare system, but they can help you navigate them more effectively, ensuring your care approaches the integration that your body naturally maintains.

The Path Forward

The evidence connecting your mouth to your overall health continues to grow stronger, making the artificial separation between dental and medical care increasingly indefensible. Progressive healthcare systems around the world have begun recognizing this reality, developing approaches that acknowledge the mouth as an integral part of the body rather than a separate domain.

In Sweden, dental care for children is connected to their overall healthcare, recognizing that early intervention can prevent both dental and systemic problems later in life. Some U.S. healthcare organizations have begun incorporating dental services, recognizing that comprehensive care reduces total healthcare costs. Forward-thinking insurance companies are experimenting with integrated dental-medical benefits, particularly for patients with chronic conditions known to have oral health connections.

These experiments in collaborative care represent the future of healthcare. One where artificial professional boundaries dissolve in favor of whole-person approaches. But you don't need to wait for system-wide change to begin experiencing more connected care.

By taking charge of your health information, insisting on communication between clinicians, and understanding the crucial interplay between oral and overall health, you can create your own microcosm of connected care.

Action Items

As you close this chapter, consider taking these immediate actions to better integrate your oral and overall healthcare:

1. **Complete a comprehensive oral-systemic assessment** at **unfaircare.com/resources**. This tool generates a personalized report identifying specific connections between your oral health and overall health conditions, providing valuable insights to share with both your dental and medical providers.

2. **Explore digital tools that facilitate dental-medical information sharing**, such as personal health record applications that can store and help you share your complete health information, including dental records, with all your doctors. As we have already discussed, the Cair app (available at Cair.net) is one such tool designed specifically for dental record management and sharing, yet it allows you to connect your medical information, too.

Implementing these targeted actions creates an integrated care approach that aligns with biological reality rather than administrative convenience.

Stop thinking of your mouth as separate from your health. Schedule your next comprehensive dental evaluation to be focused on systemic health, not just a cleaning.

Tell your healthcare providers you expect full communication across your dental, medical and specialty care.

Don't just manage your teeth. Protect your health.

THREE

Dental vs Medical—
What Each Gets Right
(and Wrong)

*"Two wrongs don't make it right, but it damn
sure makes us even."* —Kirk Jones

When Violet, a 57-year-old high school counselor, started waking up parched every morning, she blamed the dry air in her bedroom. But her discomfort soon followed her through the day, resulting in dry lips, troubled swallowing, and a sticky, metallic taste that wouldn't go away.

Violet had been managing hypertension for over a decade, faithfully taking her prescribed medications. At her annual physical, her primary care physician noted her blood pressure was well-controlled and adjusted her dosage slightly to address occasional dizziness. When Violet mentioned the persistent dry mouth, her doctor chalked it up to dehydration and told her to "just drink more water."

A few weeks later, at her routine dental check-up, Violet's hygienist noticed signs of early enamel erosion and an uptick in plaque buildup. When Violet described her dry mouth symptoms, the dentist asked about her medications. After reviewing her chart, he explained that one of her blood pressure drugs, a diuretic, was a likely the cause of her reduced saliva production. He also warned her that persistent dry mouth doesn't just feel uncomfortable, it significantly raises the risk of cavities, gum disease, and oral infections.

That visit became a turning point. Violet's dentist sent a note to her physician, suggesting alternative antihypertensives with less impact on salivary glands. The physician responded with appreciation, adjusting the prescription. Within weeks, Violet felt better. Not just in her mouth, but overall. She realized she had started sleeping better, eating more comfortably, and feeling less fatigued during the day.

Looking back, Violet was frustrated. "Why did it take so long for someone to connect the dots? I've seen my doctor and dentist regularly for years. Shouldn't they be talking to each other?"

Violet's story illustrates another example of the harm that is caused by the divide between medicine and dentistry. These two vital domains of healthcare operate in separate worlds, and failing to connect them allows avoidable problems to fester. Dry mouth isn't just an oral discomfort, it's often a symptom of systemic issues, medication side effects, or underlying conditions. When saliva production decreases, the mouth's natural defenses weaken, making patients more susceptible to infections that can affect the entire body.

Without communication between her dentist and physician, Violet would have remained caught in a cycle of discomfort and declining health. Her experience reinforces an important truth that's too often overlooked in American healthcare: oral health is not optional, cosmetic, or isolated. It is integral to your overall wellness.

The Historical Divorce

The disconnection between dentistry and medicine stems from historical accident, professional politics, and economic factors that have calcified over centuries.

In early medical history, dentistry was considered part of medicine. Hippocrates and other ancient physicians wrote extensively about oral diseases and their treatment. During the Middle Ages, however, dental care was often provided by barber-surgeons rather than physicians, beginning a separation that would widen over time.

The formal split in modern America traces back to the early 20th century. As medical education was being standardized following the influential Flexner Report of 1910, dentistry established its own separate educational system and professional organizations.

Medical schools focused increasingly on systemic diseases and hospital-based care, while dental education emphasized technical procedures centered on the mouth.

This professional separation was further reinforced when insurance systems developed after World War II. Medical insurance evolved separately from dental insurance, with different payment models, coverage limitations, and provider networks. By the time Medicare was established in 1965, the division was so entrenched that dental coverage was explicitly excluded from the program, an exclusion that largely persists today and continues to reinforce the artificial boundary between oral and systemic health.

The consequences of this historical accident are profound. This separation manifests in multiple ways, through separate records, separate doctors, separate facilities, and separate payment systems. All of which create obstacles to comprehensive, patient centered care.

Dental Strengths: What Medicine Could Learn

Despite the problems created by this separation, each system has developed strengths from which the other could learn. The dental care model, for all its limitations, excels in several areas where medical care often falls short:

1. Emphasis on Prevention

Dentistry has embraced preventive care more successfully than medicine. The standard twice-yearly cleaning and examination schedule represents a preventive approach rarely seen in medical practice.

While medical care remains largely reactive, responding to symptoms after they appear, dental care routinely incorporates scheduled preventive visits regardless of symptoms.

Dental professionals also dedicate significant time to patient education, teaching proper brushing and flossing techniques, discussing dietary choices, and emphasizing home care routines. This focus stands in stark contrast to the often rushed medical appointment where preventive counseling frequently gets shortchanged.

Jessica, a nurse practitioner, noticed this difference when comparing her medical practice with her husband's dental office: "In medicine, we talk about prevention, but our system rarely allows time for it. My husband's hygienists spend fifteen minutes per patient just on education and prevention. We're lucky if we can dedicate two minutes to preventive counseling in a typical medical visit."

The dental model's preventive emphasis extends to early intervention. Dental professionals routinely treat early-stage issues like incipient cavities or mild gingivitis before they progress to more serious conditions requiring extensive intervention. This "stitch in time" approach contrasts with medical care, where reimbursement structures and time constraints often delay intervention until conditions become more severe and expensive to treat.

2. Consistent Care Team

Dental practices typically provide continuity of care that many medical patients would envy. Patients often see the same dentist and hygienist for years or even decades, building relationships that foster trust and comprehensive understanding of the patient's history.

This continuity allows dental professionals to notice subtle changes over time. Slight recession here, minor wear patterns there. Changes that might be missed without the context of long-term observation. It also creates accountability, as doctors witness the long-term outcomes of their treatment decisions rather than passing patients to different specialists who may never communicate with each other.

When Dave, a 57-year-old teacher, developed a persistent sore throat, he cycled through four different doctors in his medical group over six months, repeating his history each time. In contrast, he's seen the same dental team for twenty years. "My dentist knows every filling in my mouth, and when it was placed. My medical visits feel like they're starting from scratch at every visit."

The dental care team model, with dentists and hygienists working collaboratively and consistently with patients, offers lessons for medical practice. While team-based care is increasingly discussed in medicine, it's been central to dental practice for decades.

The Power of a Consistent Care Team

Dentistry quietly mastered what medicine still struggles to deliver: continuity.

Patients often see the same dentist and hygienist for decades. That means subtle changes don't go unnoticed.

This isn't just convenience. It's accountability. It's context. And it's the kind of long-term, collaborative care medicine talks about, but dentistry actually delivers.

The medical world could learn a lot from the dental chair.

3. Transparent Pricing

Dental care, while far from perfect, generally offers more price transparency than medical care. Patients typically receive detailed treatment plans with associated costs before proceeding with care. This transparency allows patients to make informed financial decisions and prioritize care when necessary.

Sandra, an accountant, contrasts her experiences: "When my dentist recommended a crown, I received a detailed estimate showing exactly what I'd pay out-of-pocket. When my doctor ordered an MRI, no one could tell me what it would cost until after I received the bill, and it ended up costing me three times what I expected."

The dental model of providing relatively clear cost estimates before treatment represents a patient centered approach that medical care would do well to emulate. While dental costs remain significant barriers for many patients, at least those costs are usually predictable rather than surprising.

4. Practical Documentation

Dental records tend to be more visual, practical, and accessible than their medical counterparts. Dental charts include visual representations of teeth that allow clinicians to quickly understand a patient's status. Treatment is documented in ways that facilitate ongoing care rather than primarily serving billing purposes.

Many dental practices routinely show patients their x-rays, intraoral camera images, and charts during appointments, involving them directly in understanding their condition. This visual approach makes complex information more accessible to patients regardless of their health literacy level.

The contrast with typical medical documentation is striking. Medical records are often filled with technical language, abbreviations, and coding designed more for administrative and legal purposes than for clinical care or patient understanding. Patients rarely see their actual medical records during appointments, and accessing those records typically requires formal requests rather than being built into the care process.

Medical Strengths: What Dentistry Could Learn

While dental care excels in several areas, medical care has its own strengths that dental practice would benefit from adopting:

1. Evidence-Based Approach

Medicine has established more robust systems for evaluating evidence and translating research into clinical practice. Medical education emphasizes critical appraisal of research, and specialties develop evidence-based guidelines that are regularly updated based on new findings.

Dr. Marcus, who trained as both a physician and a dentist, notes the difference: "In medical residency, we routinely discussed recent studies and how they might change our practice. In dental settings, I've found more reliance on what doctors learned in school or what works in their experience, with less systematic integration of new evidence."

This difference appears in practice patterns as well. Medical treatments that prove ineffective are more quickly abandoned based on research evidence, while dental procedures sometimes persist based on tradition rather than outcomes data. The stronger evidence-based infrastructure in medicine, including extensive clinical trials, systematic reviews, and formal guideline development, represents a strength that dentistry would benefit from embracing more fully.

2. Holistic Assessment

Medical practice typically takes a more comprehensive view of patient health, routinely collecting information about various body systems, medications, and social factors that might influence health. The medical history and physical examination are designed to assess the patient as a whole rather than focusing on a single organ system.

This holistic approach creates opportunities to identify connections between seemingly unrelated symptoms and to address root causes rather than just treating individual manifestations. When done well, it allows for more integrated care that addresses the patient's overall health rather than isolated problems.

Dental practice, by contrast, often focuses narrowly on the mouth with limited attention to systemic conditions that might affect or be affected by oral health. Dental intake forms typically include medical history questions that are completely different from a physician's medical history, as this critical information is often treated as screening tools for contraindications, rather than as integral aspects of treatment planning.

3. Interprofessional Collaboration

While still having a long way to go, medicine has made greater strides in developing collaborative care models that integrate multiple health professionals. The concept of the care team, including physicians, nurses, pharmacists, social workers, and others working together to address complex patient needs, is increasingly common in medical settings.

This collaborative approach acknowledges that no single clinician can address all aspects of a patient's health and that different perspectives contribute to more comprehensive care. It also creates formal channels for communication among clinicians, reducing the barriers that often compromise patient care.

Dental practice, however, remains more isolated, with limited formal collaboration even among dental specialists and even less interaction with medical doctors. This isolation limits the potential for truly collaborative care and places the burden of coordination on patients themselves.

4. Accessibility Infrastructure

While far from ideal, the medical system has developed more robust infrastructure for addressing accessibility concerns. Emergency departments provide 24/7 access for acute problems. Telephone triage systems help patients determine when immediate care is needed. Hospital based care provides options for patients too ill for outpatient management.

These accessibility mechanisms, while imperfect, create safety nets that are largely absent in dental care. Dental emergencies outside of office hours often leave patients with few options beyond pain management until offices reopen. Patients requiring more intensive monitoring during dental procedures often must be referred to hospital settings that are not designed with dental care in mind.

The medical model of tiered access, from emergency care to primary care to intensive care, provides a framework that dental care could adapt to better meet patients' needs across the spectrum of acuity and complexity.

The Connection Imperative

The strengths and weaknesses of each system highlight a crucial truth: neither dental nor medical care alone provides the comprehensive, coordinated approach patients need to manage their comprehensive care. True health requires integrating the best aspects of both models while eliminating the artificial boundary between them.

This connection isn't merely a theoretical ideal. It is a practical necessity for addressing the complex health challenges patients face. For example, many medications affect oral health through side effects like dry mouth, which significantly increases cavity risk. An integrated approach would ensure that prescribing physicians consider these effects and coordinate with dentists on preventive strategies.

The benefits of integration also extend beyond clinical outcomes to include economic advantages as well. Studies consistently show that preventive dental care reduces overall healthcare costs, particularly for patients with chronic conditions. One study found that patients with diabetes who received regular dental care had 39% fewer hospital admissions and 40% lower medical costs compared to those who didn't receive dental care (Jeffcoat et al. 2014).

Making Connections Work for You

While systemic change happens slowly, you don't need to wait for healthcare reform to begin experiencing more connected care. Here are practical strategies for bridging the dental-medical divide in your own healthcare:

1. Create your own information hub

Since dental and medical systems rarely share records automatically, you can become the connection point by:

- Requesting copies of both dental and medical records
- Creating a comprehensive medication list that you share with all clinicians
- Using digital tools like the Cair app to organize and share your dental information and other information
- Maintaining a health journal that tracks symptoms that might cross the dental-medical divide

2. Facilitate cross-system communication

Don't assume your healthcare providers are communicating with each other. Make it happen by:

- Asking your dentist to send relevant findings to your physician
- Requesting your physician send health updates to your dentist
- Bringing copies of recent lab work, medication changes, or treatment plans to all appointments

Thomas, a heart patient, proactively manages this communication: "After my valve replacement, I created a one-page summary of my cardiac history, medications, and antibiotic prophylaxis requirements. I share this with my dentist and update it whenever my cardiologist makes changes. It's become my personal collaboration tool."

3. Ask integration focused questions

Prompt both medical doctors and dentists to think beyond their traditional boundaries by asking:

- "How might my medical conditions affect my dental health?"
- "Could my oral health issues be contributing to my other health problems?"
- "Should my treatments be coordinated across my healthcare team?"
- "Are any of my medications affecting my oral health?"
- "Could my dental symptoms be related to my medical conditions?"

These questions not only improve your immediate care but also help educate clinicians about the importance of collaboration, potentially benefiting their other patients as well.

4. Look for integration-oriented providers

When choosing doctors, seek those who demonstrate awareness of oral-systemic connections:

- Ask potential dentists how they incorporate patients' medical conditions into their treatment planning
- Ask potential physicians whether they include oral health assessment in their examinations
- Look for practices that have formal referral relationships across the dental-medical divide

5. Advocate for appropriate preventive coverage

Insurance systems often create barriers to connected care through arbitrary coverage limitations. Combat this by:

- Requesting "medical necessity" coverage for dental procedures related to your medical conditions
- Appealing denials with documentation of oral-systemic connections relevant to your case
- Supporting policy changes that would require medical insurance to cover dental services when oral conditions affect systemic health

Jennifer, who lives with rheumatoid arthritis, successfully advocated for her insurance to cover additional dental cleanings: "I showed them research linking periodontal disease and rheumatoid arthritis symptoms. After initial pushback, they approved coverage when my rheumatologist wrote a letter explaining how my dental care directly affected my arthritis management."

Making Connections Work For You

You don't have to wait for systemic reform to experience better connected care.

Start by collecting and sharing your records using tools like the Cair app.

Ask doctors to exchange information.

Choose doctors who value oral-systemic connections. Small actions create big improvements when you become the connector.

The Future of Connection

While individual patients can create personal workarounds, true connectivity requires systemic change. Fortunately, promising models are emerging:

Education Integration: Some universities are developing combined curricula where dental and medical students train together during portions of their education, fostering mutual understanding and collaboration habits that continue into practice.

Co-Location Models: Innovative practices are placing dental and physicians in the same physical spaces, facilitating communication and coordinated care. These range from dental hygienists working in primary care offices to comprehensive health centers offering both dental and medical services under one roof.

Digital Integration: Advanced electronic health record systems are beginning to create interoperability between both dental and medical information, creating connected patient records that support truly comprehensive care. Telehealth platforms increasingly allow for virtual consultation between dental and medical professionals.

Payment Reform: Progressive insurers are experimenting with integrated dental-medical benefits, particularly for patients with chronic conditions where oral health directly impacts overall health outcomes. These models recognize that artificial coverage divisions ultimately increase total healthcare costs.

As promising as these developments are, meaningful connection ultimately requires reimagining healthcare delivery around patients rather than professional boundaries or historical accidents. It requires shifting focus from treating diseases to maintaining health, from episodic interventions to continuous relationships, and from siloed expertise to collaborative wisdom.

Action Items

Before you learn more about your healthcare records and rights in the next chapter, consider taking these immediate actions to begin bridging the dental-medical divide in your own care:

1. **Create a provider communication matrix** mapping out which of your healthcare professionals should be sharing information with each other. Include your dentist, dental specialists, primary care physician, and medical specialists. For each connection, note what specific information would be most valuable to share (e.g., your cardiologist should know about your periodontal status, your dentist should know about your diabetes management).

2. **Draft a simple medical-dental summary**, a one-page document highlighting the key aspects of your health from both a medical and dental perspective. Include chronic conditions, medications, allergies, and recent significant health events. Keep digital and physical copies of this summary to share at appointments.

These actions begin transforming your care experience into a collaborative approach that better serves your total health needs. By actively bridging the dental-medical divide in your personal care, you not only improve your own health outcomes but also demonstrate to clinicians the value of more connected care models.

But this integration won't happen by accident. It happens only when you demand it.

The awareness of these systemic dysfunctions that you have learned is powerful, but it's only the beginning. Now, it's time to discuss how you can effectively move from outrage to ownership.

PART II

Taking Back Control

FOUR

Your Records, Your Rights

"The only people who achieve much are those
who want knowledge." —C.S. Lewis

Rachel stared at the stack of medical bills on her kitchen table, her frustration growing with each envelope she opened. After three months of persistent back pain, five doctor visits, two MRIs, and countless physical therapy sessions, she was no closer to relief.

But she was thousands of dollars poorer.

"I've told the same story to five different doctors," she sighed to her sister on the phone. "Each one orders new tests without looking at previous ones. Nobody seems to have an idea of what's happening, and I'm caught in the middle."

Her sister suggested something that hadn't occurred to Rachel, "Have you ever actually seen your medical records? Not just the summaries they hand you, but the actual notes the doctors write?"

Rachel hadn't. Like most patients, she assumed her medical records were primarily for her doctors. Technical documents written in jargon that wouldn't mean much to her anyway. When her sister explained that she had a legal right to access these records, Rachel was skeptical but desperate enough to try.

What she discovered changed everything. Upon reviewing her complete records, Rachel found critical discrepancies. Her primary doctor had documented "possible disc herniation" from her initial visit, but this detail never made it to her physical therapist. The first

MRI report mentioned "mild spinal stenosis," but this finding wasn't acknowledged in subsequent treatment plans. Most concerning, her medication allergies were inconsistently recorded, with one doctor noting an NSAID sensitivity that others had missed entirely.

Armed with her complete records, Rachel scheduled an appointment with a new spine specialist. Instead of starting from scratch, she brought organized documentation of everything that had been tried, tested, and documented. This time, the specialist quickly identified a treatment approach that had been overlooked, targeting the stenosis that previous doctors had minimized. Within weeks, Rachel experienced significant pain reduction for the first time in months.

"I wasted three months and thousands of dollars because my information was scattered across different doctors who weren't communicating," Rachel explained. "The solution was there all along, buried in records I didn't know I had a right to see."

Rachel's experience illustrates another fundamental truth of modern healthcare: **Your health records serve as the essential foundation for your healthcare empowerment.**

In this chapter, you will learn in detail the specific processes for accessing these records, the exact rights that protect your access, and strategic ways to leverage this information for superior care.

Information Segmentation

As we've already established, the disconnection between your various health records creates far more than administrative headaches. Let's examine how to overcome this imposed separation to improve your personal healthcare.

Consider these common scenarios:

- Your primary care physician prescribes a medication without knowing that your dentist has already identified an interaction risk with another drug you're taking.

- Your cardiologist makes treatment recommendations without seeing the sleep study results your pulmonologist ordered, missing the connection between your heart palpitations and undiagnosed sleep apnea.

- Your new clinic repeats expensive tests and administers additional radiographic exposures because they can't access results from your previous doctor's office.

- Your emergency room visit isn't informed by crucial information about your chronic conditions because the hospital uses a different electronic record system than your primary doctors.

These information gaps are omnipresent today and create more than just inconvenience. They result in delayed diagnoses, unnecessary procedures, dangerous medication interactions, needless radiographic exposure and wasted resources. These problems end up with the predictable result, where communication failures contribute to an estimated 30% of malpractice claims (CRICO Strategies 2015).

As we explored in Chapter 2, your oral health directly impacts your overall health, yet dental and medical records rarely communicate. This separation means your dentist might not know about your chronic kidney disease (which significantly affects oral health), while your endocrinologist remains unaware of your periodontal disease (which can make blood sugar control more difficult).

Even within single healthcare systems, information often exists in multiple separate databases. Laboratory results, imaging studies, specialist notes, pharmacy records, and billing information may all live in separate systems that communicate poorly or not at all. Electronic health records (EHRs) were supposed to solve this problem, but many have instead created digital versions of the same silos that existed on paper.

Note that the consequences of this disconnection fall primarily on you, the patient. When doctors lack complete information, you receive suboptimal care. When systems don't communicate, you bear the burden of repeating your history, coordinating your own care, and identifying contradictions or gaps that clinicians miss. And when errors occur due to missing information, you suffer the clinical and financial consequences.

🔗 Disconnected Systems, Undue Burden

When healthcare systems don't talk to each other, you become the connector.

You're the one retelling your story... again. You're the one spotting contradictions your doctor didn't see. You're the one managing referrals, reconciling meds, and chasing test results.

And when something falls through the cracks? You pay the price. In delays. In dollars. In outcomes that could have been better.

You deserve care that works together, so you don't have to hold it all together.

How to Use Upcoming Information Without Getting Overwhelmed

As we have discussed, healthcare isn't simple. And fixing your experience with your care doesn't come with a single tip or checklist. That's why the information that follows throughout this book will offer you the full spectrum; from paradigm-shifting insights to scripts, templates, and proven strategies for reclaiming control.

But you don't need to implement everything at once.

Instead, treat the remaining information in this book like a buffet. Take only what you need now. Note the tools or ideas that resonate, and trust that you can return later to the sections that speak to your next challenge.

To make implementation easier, I've curated a library of downloadable tools, templates, and quick-start guides to accompany each chapter. You can find those at **unfaircare.com/resources**. Here you will find a living, growing resource hub designed to help you take action one step at a time.

This is your healthcare revolution. Make it work for you.

Your Legal Right to Your Records

You've already discovered the first, most critical step in your journey to take command of your care: get access to all your dental and medical records.

Remember that you have legal rights to access your healthcare information, and these rights have expanded significantly in recent years. It is important for you to understand these rights, as your care team may not.

In the United States, your right to access your health information is primarily protected by two federal laws:

The Health Insurance Portability and Accountability Act (HIPAA) gives you the right to access, review, and receive copies of your medical and billing records from healthcare providers, hospitals, and health insurance companies. Under HIPAA, covered entities must provide your records within 30 days of your request (with a possible 30-day extension) and can only charge reasonable, cost based fees for providing copies.

📁 Your Right to Digital Dental Records

You have the legal right to receive your dental and medical records in digital form (which makes sense today).

Under HIPAA, if your records are stored electronically, and they should be, your provider must supply them to you electronically if you ask. Whether you want a PDF, USB copy, email, or secure app or portal access, the format must be honored if it's reasonably doable.

You don't have to accept paper if you asked for digital.

It's the law.

The 21st Century Cures Act strengthened your rights by prohibiting "Information Blocking" practices that interfere with access, exchange, or use of electronic health information. The Cures Act Final Rule, implemented in 2021, requires healthcare providers to give patients access to all electronic health information in their electronic health records "without delay".

Also, access to your information must be free of charge if it is via the patient's own system or app. This includes clinical notes, test results, dental and medical charting, medication lists, and problem lists.

Under the HIPAA Privacy Rule and the 21st Century Cures Act, healthcare providers must give patients access to their health information upon request in the form and format requested by the individual if it is readily producible in that form and format.

If the requested format isn't readily available, they must provide the records in a readable electronic form agreed upon by the patient and provider.

If you're requesting your records, you can:

- Ask if they support any mobile applications for record access
- Inquire about their secure patient portal, which may have mobile options
- Specify your preferred electronic format

These federal protections establish your baseline rights, though state laws may provide additional protections. For example, some states require faster response times, set lower fee caps, or provide special protections for sensitive information.

Despite these legal protections, many patients encounter obstacles when attempting to access their records. Healthcare organizations may:

- Impose unnecessary paperwork requirements
- Charge excessive fees
- Provide incomplete records
- Delay fulfilling requests
- Claim technical limitations
- Present information in formats that are difficult to use

These practices, while frustrating, can often be overcome with persistence and knowledge of your rights. When providers resist legitimate record requests, it's often because they're following outdated policies that haven't caught up with current regulations, not because they're legally entitled to withhold your information.

If you believe you are encountering Information Blocking, or unreasonable access to your personal health information, head over to **unfaircare.com/resources** to learn more about how to advocate for your rights and file a complaint for software vendors or healthcare providers that you believe are potentially violating these Federal mandates.

It's worth noting that there are limited exceptions to your right of access. Providers can withhold psychotherapy notes (detailed notes from mental health counseling sessions, which are different from general mental health records), information compiled for legal proceedings, and certain laboratory information. They may also deny access if they believe the information could endanger your life or physical safety. However, these exceptions are narrowly defined and don't apply to most healthcare records requests.

> ## ✋ Pause and Remember
>
> Your records aren't your doctor's property.
>
> They belong to you, by law.
>
> Claim them. Own them. Control your care.

What's Actually in Your Records

Your health records contain far more information than you might realize. Beyond the basic summary you typically receive after medical appointments, complete records include:

Clinical notes: The detailed documentation clinicians create during or after your visit, including their observations, your reported symptoms, physical examination findings, assessment of your condition, and treatment plans. These notes often contain nuanced information that never makes it into the brief summaries you typically receive.

Dental charts: Comprehensive documentation of your dental status, including tooth-by-tooth condition assessments, restoration history, missing teeth, and treatment planning notes.

Periodontal charting: Detailed measurements of gum pocket depths, recession, bleeding points, mobility, and other indicators of periodontal health that track progression or improvement of gum disease over time.

Test results: Complete laboratory reports, imaging studies, pathology results, genetic tests, and other diagnostic information. The full reports typically contain detailed technical information and the clinician's interpretation. Not just the simplified "normal/abnormal" designations you might receive automatically.

Radiographic imaging: Both medical imaging and dental x-rays including 2D (bitewings, panoramic) and 3D (cone beam CT scans) x-rays showing bone structure, tooth roots, nerve pathways, and pathology not visible during clinical examination.

Intraoral scans: Digital 3D models of your teeth and other tissues, used for treatment planning, appliance fabrication, and monitoring changes in tooth position or wear over time.

Medication records: Details of all prescribed medications, including dosages, frequencies, durations, prescribing doctors, and sometimes notes about your response or side effects.

Problem lists: The ongoing catalog of your diagnosed conditions that guides your care across visits and clinics.

Allergies and adverse reactions: Documentation of known allergies and previous adverse reactions to medications, materials, or procedures.

Immunization records: Your complete vaccination history, including dates, types, and administering clinicians.

Billing and insurance information: Detailed coding of your diagnoses, procedures, and the associated charges and payments.

Correspondence: Messages between you and your providers, as well as communication between your clinicians about your care.

This wealth of information can be intimidating, but it provides a comprehensive view of your health history that no single appointment can capture. When properly organized and understood, your complete records become a powerful tool for ensuring coordinated, appropriate care.

The depth and clinical detail in these records explain why healthcare professionals sometimes assume patients won't understand or benefit from seeing them. This paternalistic view, that healthcare information is too complex for patients to comprehend, has long been used to justify limiting patient access. However, research consistently shows that patients who access their complete records:

- Feel more in control of their care
- Better understand their health conditions
- More effectively follow treatment plans
- Identify errors and omissions that providers miss
- Ask more informed questions during appointments
- Experience less anxiety about their health (Walker et al. 2011)

As one patient advocate put it: "I may not understand every technical term in my medical record, but I certainly understand when different doctors are telling me conflicting things, or when something important about my history isn't being acknowledged."

How to Request and Organize Your Records

Accessing your complete health records requires a strategic approach. Here's a step-by-step guide to gathering and organizing this crucial information:

1. Identify all relevant providers

Start by making a comprehensive list of all healthcare professionals you've seen within the relevant timeframe (typically the last 5-10 years for chronic conditions, or 2-3 years for more recent issues). Don't forget to include:

- Primary care physicians
- Dentists and dental specialists
- Medical specialists
- Hospitals and emergency departments
- Urgent care centers
- Imaging centers
- Independent laboratories
- Mental health professionals
- Physical therapists and other rehabilitation specialists

For each professional, note their practice name, address, phone number, and the approximate dates you received care. This information will streamline your request process.

2. Submit clear, written requests

While some providers accept verbal requests for records, always submit your request electronically, or minimally in writing to create a documentation trail. Most mobile applications, like Cair, have specific forms for record requests and can automatically create this documentation trail on your behalf. If not, create your own written request that includes:

- Your full name and date of birth
- Your contact information
- The specific records you're requesting (be as specific as possible)
- The date range of records needed
- Your preferred format (secure mobile application, other electronic means or paper)
- Where to send the records (to you or to another professional)
- Your signature and the date

Be specific about what you're requesting. Rather than asking for "all my records," which might yield incomplete results, specify "all clinical notes, test results, imaging reports, medication lists, problem lists, and billing records from [date] to [date]."

For electronic records, request common formats that you can easily access, such as through a mobile application or USB drive.

3. Know your rights regarding fees

Under the 21st Century Cures Act, providers cannot charge fees for electronic access to your records through your mobile app, patient portal or similar means. For copies of electronic records delivered by other methods, they can charge only reasonable, cost-based fees for labor, supplies, and postage.

For paper records, providers can charge reasonable copying fees, typically regulated by state law. These fees often range from $0.25 to $1.00 per page, though many states cap the total amount. If you're requesting records due to financial hardship or for disability applications, mention this in your request and many clinics will reduce or waive fees in these circumstances.

If a provider attempts to charge excessive fees (such as several hundred dollars for a modest record set), politely challenge this by referencing HIPAA limitations on "reasonable, cost-based fees" and asking for a detailed breakdown of the charges.

4. Track and follow up on your requests

Record keeping is crucial when requesting health records. For each request:

- Note the date submitted
- Get the name of the person who received it
- Ask about the expected timeframe for fulfillment
- Set a calendar reminder to follow up if you haven't received a response within that timeframe

If your request is denied or ignored, escalate appropriately:

1. Contact the practice manager or health information department supervisor
2. Request to speak with the HIPAA compliance officer
3. Contact the provider's corporate headquarters if applicable
4. File a complaint with the U.S. Department of Health and Human Services Office for Civil Rights

5. Organize records effectively

As records arrive, implement a systematic organization approach. Consider these methods:

Digital organization: Create a consistent folder structure through a secure mobile app or on your computer with main folders for each provider type (e.g., Primary Care, Dental, Cardiology) and subfolders for categories like Lab Results, Imaging, Visit Notes, and Medications. Rename files with clear dates and descriptions (e.g., "2023-06-15 Bloodwork Lipid Panel").

Paper organization: Use a binder system with dividers for different healthcare professionals and categories. Consider plastic sheet protectors to prevent damage to important documents, and always keep a backup copy in a secure location.

Health record apps: Applications like the Cair app provide structured ways to organize health information, particularly dental records. Other health record apps may offer similar functionality.

Patient portals: While not a complete solution, patient portals can supplement your personally organized records by providing easy access to recent information. Just remember that portal information is typically limited and controlled by the provider.

Whichever method you choose, make sure to set aside time to incorporate new records into your system and update your health timeline as needed.

Protecting What You Own: Data Privacy Basics

Once you've accessed your health records, protecting them becomes your responsibility. These files contain highly sensitive personal information, including diagnoses, medications, mental health notes, and more. Mishandled, they can lead to identity theft, insurance discrimination, or be quietly sold to third parties.

The risk isn't just from hackers or leaks. Many apps and digital platforms are not bound by HIPAA, yet still collect and share your health data. This is especially true for free tools with vague privacy policies or business models built on advertising.

How to Protect Your Health Data

1. Encrypt Your Files
If you're storing records on your device or in the cloud, use basic encryption tools or password protection to ensure your data can't be accessed without authorization.

2. Avoid Unsecured Apps
Don't use platforms that lack clear privacy practices or fail to offer essential protections like multi-factor authentication. If the app doesn't explain how it uses your data, assume it's being shared.

3. Choose Trusted Tools
Use Personal Health Record (PHR) apps that give you control and don't resell your data. Options include:

- Cair: Built with a privacy-first approach to patient managed records. While Cair is free for most patient use, it is supported by the practices that provide it to their patients.
- Apple Health: Stores data on your device with user managed sharing.
- CommonHealth: An open source option that supports decentralized medical data access.

4. Watch for Red Flags
Avoid apps that ask for excessive permissions, don't use encryption, or partner with third-party advertisers. If a product is free and you don't know how it makes money, it's likely profiting from your data.

You've worked to gain control of your records. Don't lose that control through inattention. Protecting your information is as critical as accessing it.

Literacy: Know the Rules of the Game

If data is power, then literacy is your armor. You don't need to be a tech expert to protect yourself, but you do need to understand what's happening behind the curtain.

- **Know Your Rights:** Under HIPAA and the 21st Century Cures Act, you are entitled to access your records electronically, promptly, and without unreasonable fees. That's law, not a courtesy.
- **Read the Policies (Yes, really):** If an app says it "may share data with partners," understand that "partners" may include advertisers, insurers, or data brokers.
- **Follow the Flow:** Many "free" health tools make money by selling your data. If you're not paying with dollars, you're likely paying with access.
- **Spot Dark Patterns:** Watch for apps that nudge you into oversharing, through pre-checked boxes or confusing consent forms buried in fine print.
- **Opt Out:** Some platforms allow you to limit data use or request deletion, but they rarely make it easy. Know where to look, and don't be afraid to ask.

Owning your health data is only the first milestone. To be truly empowered, you must understand it, secure it, and decide when and how it's used.

Breaking The Code: Understanding Your Records

Medical and dental records contain specialized terminology, abbreviations, and coding systems that can seem like a foreign language to patients. While you don't need to become a medical linguist to benefit from your records, understanding a few basic principles can help you extract meaningful information.

Common abbreviations and terminology:

Healthcare professionals use hundreds of abbreviations to document efficiently. Some of the most common include:

- **Hx**: History
- **Px**: Physical examination
- **Dx**: Diagnosis
- **Rx**: Prescription or treatment
- **SOB**: Shortness of breath (not the insult!)
- **HTN**: Hypertension (high blood pressure)
- **DM**: Diabetes mellitus
- **BID**: Twice daily (medication instruction)
- **PRN**: As needed (medication instruction)
- **WNL**: Within normal limits

When encountering unfamiliar abbreviations, don't hesitate to use online medical abbreviation dictionaries or ask your healthcare professionals for clarification.

Diagnostic coding systems:

Healthcare records use standardized coding systems to classify diagnoses and procedures:

- **ICD-10** codes classify medical diagnoses. For example, E11.9 indicates Type 2 diabetes without complications.
- **CPT** codes describe procedures and services. For example, 99213 represents a moderate-complexity office visit.
- **CDT** codes specifically describe dental procedures. For example, D2150 indicates a two-surface amalgam filling.

Understanding these codes can help you verify that your diagnoses are accurately recorded and that billed procedures match what you actually received. Online code lookup tools can help you decipher specific codes in your records.

Lab and test result interpretation:

Laboratory reports typically include:

- The test name
- Your result
- The reference range (what's considered normal)
- Flags for results outside the reference range (marked as H for high or L for low)

While reference ranges are helpful guidelines, they don't tell the complete story. A value slightly outside the reference range might be normal for you, while a result within the range might still be concerning if it represents a significant change from your baseline. This is why tracking your results over time and discussing your results with the appropriate healthcare professional is so valuable.

Medication information:

Medication records should include:

- The drug name (both brand and generic)
- Dosage and form
- Administration instructions
- The condition being treated
- Start and end dates
- The prescribing doctor
- Special instructions or precautions

Pay particular attention to medication changes and note any correlations with symptom improvements or new problems. These patterns are often clearer when you review comprehensive records than when considering individual appointments in isolation.

Becoming A Medical Detective: Using Your Records

Once you've consolidated your healthcare records, you can use them to improve your care in several ways:

Identifying errors and inconsistencies:

Review your records with a critical eye, looking for:

- Factual errors in your history (incorrect dates, procedures, or family history)
- Inconsistent information across doctors
- Diagnoses that were considered but never followed up
- Recommended tests or referrals that weren't completed
- Medication discrepancies between what you're actually taking and what's documented

When you find errors, request corrections from the relevant professionals. Under HIPAA, you have the right to request amendments to inaccurate health information, though providers may deny requests they consider unfounded. Even if a formal amendment is denied, you can submit a written statement of disagreement that becomes part of your record.

Tracking patterns and connections:

Your compiled records often reveal patterns that aren't obvious during individual appointments:

- Symptoms that occur seasonally or cyclically
- Side effects that correlate with medication changes
- Gradual changes in test results that, while individually within normal ranges, show concerning trends over time
- Connections between seemingly unrelated symptoms

William, a 42-year-old engineer, suffered recurring sinus infections for years. When he reviewed his complete records, he noticed that these infections frequently occurred within weeks of dental cleanings. This observation led to the discovery of a small oral-antral communication (an opening between his mouth and sinus) that was allowing bacteria to enter his sinuses during dental procedures. Surgical repair resolved his chronic infections, illustrating the power that can come from tracking these patterns and making the right connection.

Preparing for appointments:

Use your records to create concise summaries before appointments:

- A timeline of relevant symptoms, treatments, and outcomes
- Lists of current medications and allergies
- Specific questions based on your record review
- Previous test results relevant to your current concerns

This preparation makes appointments more productive and prevents the common scenario where patients remember critical details only after leaving the doctor's office.

Bring more than just yourself to your next appointment. Bring clarity, using your records to create a 1-page prep sheet that includes your symptoms, treatments, and outcomes and specific questions to ask your doctor.

This simple act transforms your visit from a vague conversation into a focused collaboration.

Don't remember what matters on the drive home. Have it in hand when it counts.

Facilitating second opinions:

When seeking second opinions, comprehensive records prevent time consuming and expensive repetition of tests. They also ensure the consulting professional has complete information rather than relying solely on your recollection or the referring doctor's summary.

Margaret, a 56-year-old with chronic joint pain, had seen four specialists who offered different diagnoses ranging from fibromyalgia to early rheumatoid arthritis. Before seeing a fifth specialist, she organized her complete records and identified conflicting test interpretations. The new rheumatologist, with access to all previous data, recognized a pattern consistent with seronegative spondyloarthritis, a condition that explained her symptoms but had been missed by doctors seeing only partial information.

Coordinating care across doctors:

Perhaps most importantly, your organized records can bridge the gaps between disparate healthcare systems:

- Share dental records with physicians when relevant (and vice versa)
- Ensure specialists are aware of all your medications and conditions
- Prevent redundant testing and radiographs by providing recent results
- Identify conflicting treatment recommendations that require resolution

By becoming the information hub for your own care, you compensate for the system's failure to coordinate effectively.

Medical and Dental Record Connection: The Missing Link

As discussed in Chapter 3, the separation between medical and dental care represents a particularly harmful fragmentation of healthcare information. Uniting this rift is crucial for truly comprehensive care.

This integration is so important that it deserves special attention within your record gathering strategy. Specifically:

1. **Request complete dental records**, including:
   › Dental charting
   › Periodontal charting (measurements of gum health)
   › Full treatment history
   › Upcoming treatment plans
   › Dental radiographs (x-rays)
   › Clinical notes documenting oral conditions

2. **Share relevant dental information with medical professionals**, particularly regarding:
   › Periodontal disease status (given its connections to diabetes, heart disease, and other conditions)
   › Oral infections or inflammation (including lumps, bumps and sores)
   › Sleep apnea evaluations or treatments
   › TMJ disorders that might relate to headaches or other symptoms
   › Medications prescribed by dentists

3. **Similarly, share pertinent medical information with dentists**, especially:
   › Diabetes status and recent A1c levels
   › Cardiovascular conditions requiring antibiotic prophylaxis
   › Osteoporosis treatments that might affect dental procedures
   › Immunosuppressive medications
   › Pregnancy status

This cross-domain information sharing often reveals connections that individual doctors might miss.

The Cair app, mentioned in previous chapters, can be particularly valuable for this integration. By digitizing and organizing your dental information in an accessible format, it facilitates sharing crucial oral health data with physicians who might otherwise remain unaware of significant findings.

The Future of Health Information Access

The landscape of health information access is evolving rapidly. New technologies and regulations are expanding patients' ability to access, understand, and utilize their healthcare data.

Interoperability initiatives aim to enable different electronic health record systems to communicate effectively. Federal rules increasingly require healthcare organizations to implement standardized data exchange capabilities, though progress remains inconsistent.

Patient centered data platforms are emerging to aggregate information from multiple doctors into unified personal health records. These platforms range from smartphone apps to sophisticated online services that can integrate data from wearable devices, patient reported outcomes, and traditional medical records.

OpenNotes and similar transparency movements promote real-time patient access to the notes doctors write during appointments. Research shows that when patients can review these notes, they better understand their conditions, more faithfully follow treatment plans, and identify errors that providers miss (DesRoches et al. 2019).

Artificial Intelligence (AI) tools are beginning to help patients interpret complex medical information, identify patterns in their health data, and prepare more effectively for healthcare encounters.

While these developments hold promise, they remain unevenly implemented. The reality is that for the foreseeable future, patients who want comprehensive access to their health information will need to be proactive rather than waiting for perfect systemic solutions.

Action Items

As you prepare to explore the quagmire of healthcare economics in the next chapter, consider taking these immediate actions to gain control of your health information:

1. **Submit record requests** to your most important healthcare professionals using the template available at **unfaircare.com /resources**. This template incorporates language specifically designed to overcome common obstacles to record access.

2. **Create a medication list** that includes all prescription drugs, over-the-counter medications, and supplements you currently take. Include dosages, frequencies, start dates, and the conditions each is treating. Share this list with all your providers at every visit.

These actions establish the foundation for what you will explore next: how money flows through the healthcare system, how these financial currents influence your care, and how understanding these dynamics can help you make more informed healthcare decisions.

By taking control of your health information, you've already begun shifting the power balance in your favor. You're not just a recipient of healthcare anymore. You are becoming an informed, active participant in your own care. This transformation represents the first essential step toward getting the quality care you deserve in a system that often seems designed to prevent exactly that.

Remember, your data is your power. Stop waiting for permission and claim it now.

FIVE

Follow the Money

"It's funny how money changes a situation." —Lauryn Hill

Mark's hands trembled slightly as he tore open the envelope from the hospital. His stomach twisted when he saw the number printed at the top: $14,783.

His first thought was that it must be a mistake. "A couple hours in the ER couldn't possibly cost that much", he reasoned, blinking rapidly as if the numbers might rearrange themselves into something more reasonable.

Heart pounding, he grabbed his phone and immediately called his wife. "They charged us almost fifteen grand," he said, voice tight with disbelief. "For a few injections and a couple hours of sitting around."

After the initial shock wore off, Mark, a financial analyst by profession, switched into problem-solving mode. He wasn't the kind of person to blindly pay a bill he didn't understand. After a deep breath, he called and requested an itemized bill from the hospital's billing department, steeling himself for the fight he suspected was coming.

When the itemized statement arrived a week later, it was even worse than he feared:

- Emergency room level 4 visit: $3,875
- Physician services: $1,258
- Epinephrine injection: $725
- IV administration: $987

- Pharmacy services: $1,440
- Observation services: $2,100
- Laboratory tests: $2,850
- Facility fee: $1,548

Mark spent the next few evenings meticulously preparing for the certain battle that was to come. Using his medical records (as discussed in Chapter 4) and online resources like Healthcare Bluebook and Medicare reimbursement rates, he compiled evidence.

He flagged multiple lab tests that weren't documented in his records, and found that a reasonable price of the epinephrine he received was closer to $15, not $725. He also printed screenshots showing typical ER visit charges in his area, which were a fraction of what he had been billed.

Armed with a binder full of research, Mark called the hospital billing department.

"Hi, this is Mark Taylor. I'm calling about a bill that appears to have multiple discrepancies," he began, keeping his voice steady.

There was a long pause on the other end of the line.

"Um, can you be more specific?" the representative finally asked.

"Sure. First, the lab tests listed were never performed according to my medical records. Second, the pharmacy charges include medications I never received. And third, the cost for the epinephrine injection is about 5,000% higher than market value. I have documentation for all of this."

What followed were days of tense, yet tedious conversations, each one requiring patience, persistence, and an unwavering attention to detail. Every time a representative tried to dismiss his concerns, Mark calmly referenced specific records. When his case escalated to a billing supervisor, he was ready.

At one point, an exasperated supervisor said, "Well, these charges are standard."

Mark didn't flinch.

"Standard doesn't mean correct," he replied evenly. "I'm asking for the charges to reflect the actual services provided, based on documented care."

Eventually, his persistence paid off. The hospital reduced his bill to $3,241. Still painful, but less than a quarter of the original amount. The billing supervisor sheepishly admitted that "coding errors" had led to the inflated charges, while insisting it was "an isolated incident."

But, was it really? Studies show that up to 80% of medical bills contain errors, and those errors rarely benefit the patient (Gooch 2016).

Reflecting on the experience later, Mark said, "The system counted on me being too intimidated, confused, or busy to question these charges. I won only because I had the skills, time, and stubbornness to fight back. But what about everyone who can't?"

The ordeal permanently changed his approach to healthcare. Now, Mark requests itemized bills upfront, researches estimated costs before procedures, and refuses to accept vague billing explanations. He even teaches family and friends how to advocate for themselves, arming them with tools he wished he had before that first shock came in the mail.

Mark's journey from stunned disbelief to decisive action highlights a fundamental truth; to navigate healthcare effectively, you must understand how money flows through the system. This knowledge isn't just about saving dollars. It's about reclaiming agency over your care in a system designed to overwhelm and outlast you.

It's not a mystery why the system is broken. What appears on the surface to be a healthcare failure is often a financial success for someone. To understand how deeply this misalignment runs, we must first examine the incentives baked into the foundation of care delivery.

The Incentives Trap

To understand why healthcare fails so consistently, follow the money.

Clinics earn more by seeing more patients and ordering more procedures, not by keeping people healthy or providing excellent outcomes. This creates an incentive structure where your doctor makes more money when you're sick than when you're well.

A dentist colleague once confided: "I know preventive care is better for patients, but I can't keep my practice open just doing check-ups and discussing peoples' sugar consumption. I need fillings and crowns to pay the bills." His honesty was refreshing, but his dilemma reveals a core problem in our system: healthcare professionals are trapped in a system that, in many instances, financially punishes them for doing what's best for patients.

🪤 Trapped by the System

Imagine being a healthcare professional who wants to prevent illness, but gets paid only when you are sick.

This is the quiet reality for many doctors. The system doesn't reward the right care, it rewards the reimbursable care. Until that changes, doctors will remain financially penalized for keeping people healthy.

Meanwhile, insurance companies profit by collecting premiums and minimizing payouts. Their financial interest lies in denying claims, not in facilitating care. Administrative staff at both insurance companies and healthcare facilities spend countless hours arguing over coverage rather than improving patient outcomes.

The result? The U.S. spends twice as much on healthcare administration as other developed nations, and all these additional costs deliver zero clinical benefit to patients (Himmelstein et al. 2020).

Pharmaceutical companies and medical device manufacturers further complicate matters, aggressively marketing directly to consumers and healthcare professionals alike. Their goal isn't necessarily to improve health outcomes but to increase market share and profits. The pharmaceutical industry spends nearly twice as much on marketing as on research and development, a shocking, yet telling statistic about their priorities (Schwartz and Woloshin 2019).

This malalignment creates a perfect storm where every major

player in healthcare benefits financially from complexity, opacity, and often, your continued illness rather than your sustained wellness.

The consequences of this incentives trap extend far beyond financial waste. They directly impact clinical decisions and patient outcomes.

Consider the case of back pain, one of the most common health complaints in America. Evidence shows that for most uncomplicated back pain, conservative approaches like physical therapy, appropriate exercise, and time are most effective. Yet many patients are quickly channeled toward expensive imaging, specialist consultations, invasive injections, and even surgery. These are interventions that often provide no better outcomes but generate significantly more revenue (Deyo et al. 2009).

A revealing study found that when physicians own MRI equipment, their patients are significantly more likely to receive MRI scans, regardless of clinical necessity (Mitchell 2008). This isn't because these physicians are malicious or unethical; it's because the system has aligned a financial reward system with more intervention rather than better outcomes.

This problematic financial structuring is equally evident in pharmaceutical prescribing patterns. When pharmaceutical representatives provide meals, speaking fees, or other "educational" benefits to physicians, those physicians prescribe more of that company's medications, even when cheaper, equally effective alternatives exist. Again, this isn't necessarily due to a conscious bias but to the subtle influence of rewards that prioritize corporate profits over patient wellbeing.

Perhaps most concerning is how the misaligned system affects end-of-life care. The fee-for-service model encourages aggressive interventions even when they provide minimal benefit and significant suffering. Patients often receive costly, invasive treatments in their final months that don't align with their personal values or wishes. However, these procedures are performed simply because the system financially rewards intervention over compassion.

These stories aren't outliers. And until we change our incentives, even the best-intentioned doctors will remain trapped in a system that is designed to work against their patients.

The Economics of Incentives

Unlike most industries where consumer choice drives competition, healthcare employs exceptionally complex economic mechanics. These specialized financial structures require equally specialized navigation techniques, which you will explore throughout this chapter.

Third-party Distortion

The presence of health insurance, while necessary for financial protection in the United States, fundamentally distorts healthcare economics. Unlike almost any other service you purchase, in healthcare:

1. The person receiving the service (you) rarely knows the actual price beforehand
2. The person providing the service (your doctor) often doesn't know the price either
3. The person primarily paying for the service (the insurer) isn't the one receiving it
4. The price for identical services varies wildly depending on who's paying

This system creates a disconnection between cost and value that would be considered absurd in other contexts. Imagine buying groceries without prices displayed, having a third-party negotiate different rates for each food item based on your employer, and receiving a bill weeks later for amounts you never agreed to. The grocery industry would collapse under such a model, yet this is exactly how healthcare typically operates.

The consequences of this distortion extend far beyond confusion. When patients are insulated from direct costs, and healthcare professionals are rewarded based on volume rather than outcomes, the result is predictable: more services delivered, regardless of necessity or value.

The net result? A 2019 study estimated that 25-30% of all healthcare spending, approximately $760-910 billion annually, goes to services that provide no clinical benefit to patients (Shrank et al. 2019).

Fee-for-Service: Paying for Volume Over Value

Most healthcare, including dental care, in America operates under a fee-for-service model, where clinicians are paid for each service rendered rather than for successful outcomes. This creates an obvious bonus structure: more services generate more revenue, regardless of whether those services improve patient health.

These patterns don't necessarily reflect conscious decisions to provide unnecessary care. Rather, they demonstrate how finances unconsciously shape clinical judgment. When the system rewards intervention over restraint, even well intentioned healthcare professionals drift toward doing more rather than doing better.

Dr. Emily Crane, an internal medicine physician, described this pressure; "I know the evidence shows most uncomplicated back pain resolves without imaging. But when patients expect something to be 'done,' ordering an MRI takes less time than explaining why it's unnecessary and generates revenue rather than costs it. The incentives all push in one direction. Fighting against that current every day is exhausting."

The fee-for-service model particularly disadvantages preventive care, which typically generates minimal immediate revenue while potentially reducing future services. A healthcare system truly designed around patient wellness would heavily incentivize prevention. Ours does the opposite, rewarding doctors financially for treating preventable conditions after they develop rather than preventing them in the first place.

The Insurance Labyrinth

Health insurers profit by collecting more in premiums than they pay out in claims, creating a fundamental tension with their stated purpose of financing healthcare.

This tension manifests in multiple ways:

- **Administrative burden**: Complex prior authorization requirements, documentation demands, and claims processes aren't accidental inefficiencies, they deliberately create friction that discourages care (Cutler 2021). If a percentage of providers abandon legitimate claims due to bureaucratic obstacles, insurers benefit financially.

- **Narrow networks**: Limiting patients to specific providers allows insurers to negotiate lower rates but often separates patients from doctors they trust and forces them to restart care relationships.

- **Coverage gaps**: The fine print of insurance policies often excludes services that would benefit patients but cost insurers, particularly in categories like mental health and restorative dental care.

- **High deductibles**: The trend toward high deductible health plans shifts costs to patients, who often avoid necessary preventive care to save money, ultimately resulting in more expensive treatments later.

Jennifer, a human resources director with twenty years of experience, summarized the situation bluntly: "Insurance isn't designed to optimize your care. It is designed to predict and limit financial risk for the insurer. The moment you forget that, you're at a disadvantage."

Pricing Opacity

Perhaps the most obvious symptom of healthcare's broken economics is the deliberate concealment of prices until after services are delivered, a practice that would be considered fraudulent in virtually any other industry, as we have already discussed.

However this problem is more pervasive than most realize. Take, for example, the fact that most hospitals maintain "chargemasters". These are comprehensive lists of prices for every service and supply they offer, where these prices bear little relationship to actual costs, what insurers pay, or what the market would support with transparent competition. Instead, they serve as artificially inflated starting points for negotiations with insurers and as the basis for bills sent to uninsured patients.

The disconnect between chargemaster rates and reality can be staggering:

- A hospital might charge $18 for a single acetaminophen tablet that costs less than $0.05 retail
- A basic blood test that costs $20 at an independent laboratory might be billed at $300 in a hospital setting
- An MRI that costs $350 at a standalone imaging center might be charged at $3,500 by a hospital

These inflated charges aren't meant to be paid in full by most patients. They are, instead, primarily negotiating anchors that make the discounted rates given to insurers seem reasonable by comparison. But for uninsured patients or those seeking care outside their insurance networks, these fictional prices become very real financial burdens.

> **80% of hospital bills contain errors, almost always in the hospital's favor.**
>
> (Medical Billing Advocates of America 2014)

The Negotiated Rate Secret

Even when hospitals and providers have established contracted rates with insurers, these rates typically remain hidden from patients until after services are delivered. This opacity eliminates price competition and enables dramatic variations in cost for identical services, often within the same geographic area or even the same facility.

Studies consistently show that prices for common procedures can vary by 500% or more among clinics in the same city, with no correlation to quality measures (Mehrotra et al. 2017). A knee replacement might cost $24,000 at one hospital and $75,000 at another ten miles away, with no difference in clinical outcomes.

This variation exists not because of differences in care quality or clinic costs, but because each insurer negotiates separate rates with each provider. These negotiations are conducted behind closed doors without consumer input or awareness. The result is a system where neither patients nor doctors have the information necessary to make value-based decisions.

The Hospital Price Transparency Rule, implemented in 2021, theoretically required hospitals to publish their negotiated rates. But compliance has been inconsistent, and even when available, this information remains difficult for the average patient to interpret or use effectively before receiving care.

Following the Money Trail in Dental Care

The economics of dental care present both parallels and contrasts to medical economics. Understanding these patterns can help you navigate both systems more effectively.

Insurance That Isn't Insurance

Dental insurance differs fundamentally from medical insurance. While medical insurance provides meaningful financial protection against catastrophic costs, dental "insurance" functions more like a prepaid discount plan with significant limitations:

- Annual coverage limits typically range from $1,000 to $2,000, an amount that hasn't increased meaningfully since the 1970s despite substantial inflation in dental costs
- Preventive services are usually covered at 100%, basic restorative at 80%, and major procedures at only 50%
- Many procedures, including implants and some specialized treatments, are typically excluded entirely
- Waiting periods often delay coverage for anything beyond basic preventive care

These limitations mean that dental insurance helps most with inexpensive preventive care but provides minimal protection against major dental expenses.

This is exactly the opposite of how insurance should function.

This coverage gap creates perverse motivations for both patients and doctors. Patients often pursue only the care their insurance covers, even when other treatments would provide better long term outcomes. Doctors feel pressure to modify treatment plans to maximize insurance reimbursement rather than optimizing patient health.

Dr. Gary, a prosthodontist who specializes in complex dental reconstruction, described this challenge, "I regularly see patients who need comprehensive treatment but have postponed care until serious problems develop because their insurance wouldn't cover earlier intervention. By the time they reach me, both the clinical challenges and the costs have multiplied significantly, and their insurance still covers only a fraction of what's needed."

The Fee Schedule Squeeze

Dentists who participate with insurance plans agree to fixed fee schedules that typically pay significantly less than their standard rates. While insurance companies justify these reduced rates by promising increased patient volume, the financial strain introduces several problematic dynamics.

To remain viable, practices must see more patients in less time, which inevitably reduces the time available for each patient. This pressure can lead to an unconscious prioritization of procedures that offer more favorable reimbursement relative to the time they take. As a result, comprehensive treatment approaches, those that address root causes rather than just symptoms, become financially challenging to sustain.

These dynamics help explain why dental appointments often feel rushed, why care may focus on immediate issues instead of long-term prevention, and why healthcare professionals may feel compelled to recommend more aggressive procedures than are absolutely necessary.

Understanding these dynamics doesn't mean your dentist is deliberately providing suboptimal care. Rather, it reveals how financial structures shape practice patterns in ways that don't always align with patient interests.

If you have questions about your care, a second opinion is always a good idea. Either through seeing another doctor, or obtaining your information through a mobile application, like Cair, which can allow you to leverage tools that screen treatment recommendations and ensure that you are aligned with your care team's suggestions.

The Cash Discount Reality

A growing number of dental practices offer significant discounts for patients who pay cash rather than using insurance. These discounts, often 20-30% off standard rates, reflect the administrative burden insurance creates and the delay in payment providers experience when billing third parties.

This practice reveals an important truth; the "insurance benefit" may sometimes be less valuable than the savings available by bypassing insurance entirely, especially for routine care or when approaching annual coverage limits.

Hospital Economics: The Inpatient Revenue Machine

Hospital care represents the most expensive component of healthcare, consuming approximately 33% of all healthcare spending (CMS 2023). Understanding hospital economics is therefore crucial to successfully navigate the healthcare landscape.

Hospital Payment Incentives

Bundled Payments and Classification Games: Hospitals operate under payment systems that can compromise patient care. Under Diagnosis Related Groups (DRGs), hospitals receive fixed payments regardless of actual services provided, incentivizing quick discharges and potentially viewing complex patients as financial burdens. Meanwhile, the arbitrary distinction between "inpatient" and "observation" status can dramatically affect both patient costs and hospital reimbursement, often based on documentation details rather than actual care needs.

These help explain why hospital discharges sometimes feel premature and why comprehensive care coordination often falls short during the critical transition from hospital to home.

Facility Fees: When hospitals acquire physician practices, they typically add "facility fees" that can double or triple costs without changing locations, providers, or services, and without providing additional value to patients (Health Care Cost Institute 2023). These fees represent revenue capture through hospital market power rather than improved care quality, making independent providers often more cost-effective for routine services.

Pharmaceutical Industry Practices That Increase Costs

Prescription drug costs represent another area where financial interests frequently override wellness, particularly in the United States, which pays substantially higher prices than other developed nations for identical medications.

The Research and Development Myth

Pharmaceutical companies often justify high drug prices by claiming they are essential to fund the research and development of new medications. While there is some truth to this narrative, it obscures several important realities. In practice, major pharmaceutical firms typically allocate significantly more of their budgets to marketing than to research and development (Schwartz and Woloshin 2019).

Furthermore, many groundbreaking drugs originate not within corporate labs, but from publicly funded research conducted at universities and government institutions. Adding to the complexity, the most expensive drugs on the market are frequently not entirely novel treatments, but rather incremental refinements of existing medications.

This doesn't mean pharmaceutical innovation isn't expensive or valuable. But the direct connection between current high prices and future medical advances is far more tenuous than industry marketing suggests.

The Pharmacy Benefit Manager Puzzle

Pharmacy Benefit Managers (PBMs), who are middlemen that administer prescription drug programs for insurers, add another layer of complexity and cost to medication economics. PBMs negotiate discounts and rebates from drug manufacturers but often don't pass these savings to patients or insurers.

This system creates the absurd structure where PBMs may prefer higher priced drugs that offer larger rebates over lower priced alternatives that would cost patients and insurers less overall. The result is a market that drives prices up rather than down, contrary to normal economic principles.

⚠️ **Step Therapy: Medicine by Trial and Error**

Imagine your doctor prescribes the medication best suited for you, but your insurance demands you first fail on cheaper, older drugs.

This is step therapy in action: insurers forcing patients to start with lower-cost treatments, even when they are less effective or inappropriate.

The goal isn't better health. It's lower short-term costs, no matter how much suffering, delay, or complication it causes.

When PBM's and insurers design the care pathway, patients are stuck playing medical roulette.

Generic Delays and Patent Games

Pharmaceutical companies use a range of strategies to extend patent protection and delay the arrival of generic competition, thereby preserving their market exclusivity and profit margins.

One common tactic is "evergreening," which involves making minor modifications to existing drugs, such as altering dosage forms or delivery mechanisms, to secure new patents.

Companies also frequently file multiple overlapping patents on various aspects of a single drug, creating legal thickets that are difficult and costly for generics to navigate. In some cases, brand-name manufacturers engage in "pay-for-delay" agreements, compensating generic drug makers to postpone their market entry. Additionally, they may introduce "authorized generics", generic versions of their own drugs, to retain control over the lower-cost segment of the market.

Collectively, these strategies can extend profit-generating monopolies for years beyond the expiration of the original patent, driving up costs for patients and insurers without delivering corresponding improvements in therapeutic value.

Strategies for Financial Self-Defense

Understanding these healthcare economics isn't just academic, it leads to practical tools you can use to protect yourself financially while obtaining quality care. Here are specific strategies for navigating each segment of the healthcare system:

Seek Doctors Who Seek Financial Clarity

An increasing number of healthcare professionals recognize the dysfunction of current healthcare economics and offer transparent, straightforward pricing. These might include:

- Direct primary care practices that charge monthly membership fees instead of per-visit charges
- Cash based specialists who publish their prices and don't contract with insurance
- Surgery centers that offer bundled pricing for procedures
- Dental practices with membership plans that replace traditional insurance

These providers typically deliver equal or better care at lower total costs by eliminating administrative overhead and aligning their goals directly with patient wellbeing rather than third-party payers.

Jason found this approach transformative for his family's healthcare: "We pay $150 monthly for our direct care membership covering our family of four. Our physician spends 45 minutes on visits, answers texts directly, and has negotiated discounted rates for labs and medications. Even with a high deductible insurance plan for emergencies, we're saving money while receiving better care."

Similarly, Emma's experience with her family's dental care shifted dramatically when her dentist introduced a membership plan through DentalHQ: "Our family pays a relatively low fee monthly for our dental membership plan. The value is incredible. We all get two cleanings yearly, all necessary X-rays, and a significant discount on additional treatments. Our dentist spends more time with us during appointments, and the office team members know us by name. The best part is how transparent the pricing is, with no insurance surprises or waiting periods. When my daughter needed a filling, I knew exactly what it would cost with our membership discount. The membership has completely changed how we think about dental visits."

Price Shopping: When and How

For nonurgent, scheduled services, price comparisons can yield substantial savings. Effective price shopping requires:

1. Getting the specific CPT or CDT codes for the services you need
2. Contacting multiple clinics for their cash price and insurance negotiated rates
3. Checking quality metrics to ensure you're comparing equivalent services
4. Considering the full episode of care, not just individual components

This approach is especially effective when applied to services that are typically planned in advance and allow for price transparency and comparison. It works particularly well for imaging studies such as MRIs, CT scans, and ultrasounds, as well as laboratory testing, dental procedures, and scheduled surgeries.

Many insurers and electronic platforms now offer price comparison tools, though their accuracy and completeness vary significantly.

Understanding EOBs and Medical Bills

The Explanation of Benefits (EOB) statements from your insurer and the bills you receive from clinics also contain important information for financial self-defense:

- **Match services received to services billed.** Using the medical records you've obtained (as discussed in Chapter 4), verify that you're only being billed for services actually provided.

- **Compare the provider's billed amount with the insurer's allowed amount.** The difference represents the "discount" negotiated by your insurance, one measure of its value to you.

- **Check for duplicate billing.** Hospitals sometimes bill separately for services that should be bundled together.

- **Verify correct coding.** Providers may inadvertently use incorrect codes that result in higher charges or reduced insurance coverage.

- **Appeal inappropriate denials.** Insurers sometimes reject legitimate claims based on technicalities or miscoded information.

When reviewing bills, remember that healthcare providers typically accept prompt payment as justification for significant discounts. Always ask: "If I pay today, can you offer a discount?" Discounts of up to 30% for immediate payment are not uncommon, particularly for larger bills.

Using Tax-Advantaged Accounts Strategically

Several account types allow you to pay for healthcare with pretax dollars, effectively discounting all your medical expenses by your tax rate:

- **Health Savings Accounts (HSAs)** offer the greatest tax advantage, with tax free contributions, growth, and withdrawals for qualified expenses. However, these are typically only available with eligible high deductible health plans.

- **Flexible Spending Accounts (FSAs)** provide tax-free funds for healthcare expenses but usually require funds to be used within the plan year.

- **Health Reimbursement Arrangements (HRAs)** are employer funded accounts that reimburse qualified medical expenses.

Strategic use of these accounts requires understanding their different rules and limitations. The key principle is maximizing tax advantaged funding while ensuring you can access the funds when needed for healthcare expenses.

Negotiating Healthcare

Many patients don't realize that healthcare costs may be negotiable in many cases, sometimes dramatically so. Effective negotiation requires understanding both the provider's economics and your leverage points.

Hospital Bill Negotiation

For substantial hospital bills, consider these approaches:

1. **Request itemized billing.** Hospitals often reduce charges when forced to justify each line item.

2. **Identify errors and duplications.** As previously mentioned, studies suggest up to 80% of hospital bills contain errors, most favoring the hospital (Gooch 2016).

3. **Compare charges to Medicare rates.** While you won't pay Medicare prices as a private patient, knowing that the government pays approximately 40% of billed charges provides negotiating context (Anderson 2007).

4. **Offer cash settlement.** Some hospitals will accept immediate payment of 60-70% of billed charges rather than pursuing full payment through extended collection efforts.

5. **Request charity care consideration.** Most nonprofit hospitals have financial assistance programs with sliding scales that extend well into middle income ranges.

Elena successfully used these techniques after an emergency appendectomy resulted in a $23,000 bill, "I requested itemized billing, identified three procedures I never received, researched Medicare rates for the legitimate services, and offered to settle immediately for 65% of the corrected amount. After some back-and-forth, they accepted my offer, saving me nearly $11,000."

Prescription Drug Strategies

Medication costs can often be reduced through:

1. **Requesting generic alternatives** whenever possible
2. **Using prescription discount cards or apps** like GoodRx, which often provide better prices than insurance copays
3. **Comparing prices across pharmacies,** which can vary substantially for identical medications
4. **Asking for 90-day supplies,** which typically cost less per day than 30-day prescriptions
5. **Exploring patient assistance programs** offered by pharmaceutical manufacturers

These approaches require active involvement and sometimes challenging conversations with doctors and pharmacists, but the financial benefits can be substantial, particularly for ongoing medications.

The Price Transparency Movement

After decades of deliberate opacity, healthcare is experiencing the early stages of a price transparency revolution. Federal regulations now require both hospitals and insurers to publish their prices, though implementation remains inconsistent and the resulting data often proves difficult for average consumers to interpret.

This movement represents a significant opportunity for patients willing to engage with financial information before receiving care. When combined with quality data, price transparency enables value-based healthcare decisions that were previously impossible.

Supporting this movement requires not just using available price information but actively demanding transparency when it's absent. Every time you ask "How much will this cost?" before receiving care, you contribute to this important culture shift toward financial clarity in healthcare.

> ## 📢 A Simple Question That Changes Everything
>
> Every time you ask, "How much will this cost?" before agreeing to treatment, you're doing more than protecting your wallet.
>
> You're forcing a broken system to face a basic expectation: financial honesty.
>
> One question. One patient at a time. One culture shift underway.

Action Items

As you get ready to explore strategies for hacking better care in the next chapter, consider taking these immediate actions to improve your healthcare financial literacy:

1. **Request an itemized bill** for your most recent significant healthcare expense. Compare it with your medical records and insurance EOB to identify any discrepancies.

2. **Research transparent pricing options** in your area for both medical and dental care. This might include direct primary care practices, cash based specialists, or dental membership plans that bypass traditional insurance.

Understanding the financial currents that shape healthcare doesn't just save you money, it fundamentally changes your relationship with the healthcare system and places pressure to ultimately create much needed systemic change. When you recognize the economic forces driving clinical decisions, you can more effectively advocate for care that truly serves your needs rather than the system's financial benefit.

The financial insights you've developed provide essential context for our next chapter, where you will learn to implement tactical approaches to overcome administrative barriers and secure optimal care.

Money may drive much of healthcare, but by leveraging knowledge you have the power to redirect its flow toward better care for yourself and, ultimately, for all.

Before you pay another healthcare bill blindly, demand an itemized statement, audit it yourself and challenge inaccuracies. If you don't defend your wallet, nobody will.

Healthcare profits from your silence. Speak up.

SIX

How to Hack Better Care

"Every action you take is a vote for the type of
person you wish to become." —James Clear

When Sophia, a 34-year-old police officer, was diagnosed with an autoimmune condition, she quickly discovered that traditional healthcare wouldn't provide the coordinated care she needed. After three specialists gave contradictory advice and her symptoms worsened despite medication, she decided to take control.

"I realized I needed to manage the system rather than follow it," she explained. "The traditional model wasn't designed for someone like me with a complex, chronic condition that crosses multiple specialties."

Sophia began by gathering her complete medical records and creating detailed spreadsheets tracking her symptoms, medications, diet, sleep patterns, and stress levels. She researched her condition extensively, joining patient communities and reading medical journal articles. When meeting with new doctors, she arrived with organized summaries of her history, current treatments, and specific questions based on her research.

"The dynamic completely changed," she recalled. "Instead of being a passive receiver of convoluted care, I became the coordinator of my own care team. I greatly respected my doctors' expertise, but I stopped expecting the system to connect the dots for me."

Sophia found a primary care physician willing to be her "medical home base" and collaborate with her proactive approach. She received copies of all correspondence between doctors and learned to interpret her own lab results. She found an integrative medicine practitioner to address lifestyle factors her specialists rarely discussed, and coordinated dental appointments with her medication schedule to minimize inflammation.

Within eight months, Sophia's symptoms had improved significantly, and she required less medication than initially prescribed. Perhaps more importantly, she no longer felt helpless against her condition or frustrated by the healthcare system.

"I didn't change my medical condition, but I completely changed my relationship to it and to healthcare. I learned to work around the system's flaws rather than being victimized by them."

Sophia's experience illustrates what this chapter is all about; practical strategies for navigating better care from an imperfect system. While systemic healthcare reform remains necessary, you don't need to wait for policy changes to improve your personal care experience.

The Mindset Shift: From Patient to CEO

A critical step in creating better care for yourself is developing a fundamental shift in how you view your role within the healthcare system. Traditional models cast you as a passive "patient." Literally defining you as someone who waits and endures.

Effective healthcare hacking requires rejecting this passive role in favor of becoming the Chief Executive Officer of your own health.

In your new healthcare leadership role, you'll move beyond accepting default offerings to actively designing your care. You will:

- **Set the vision and strategy for your care**, determining priorities and desired outcomes rather than simply accepting whatever the system offers

- **Assemble and manage your care team**, selecting healthcare professionals who meet your standards rather than accepting random assignments

- **Coordinate communication and operations** between different components of your healthcare

- **Evaluate performance and results**, holding professionals accountable for both clinical outcomes and service quality

This mindset shift doesn't mean disrespecting healthcare professionals or their expertise. Rather, it means recognizing that even the most excellent doctors are operating within a broken system that doesn't naturally promote coordination, prevention, or personalization. By assuming executive responsibility for your care, you create connection where the system creates fragmentation.

Seek to become the most effective CEO of your health you can be. Successful leaders recognize that they are likely not the expert in any specific area under their governance, but rather they set the vision and select the best experts for the team.

Frank, a 58-year-old construction worker who successfully navigated treatment for prostate cancer, described this mindset shift: "I approached my diagnosis like a complex project requiring management. My doctors were vital team members with specialized knowledge, but I was the project manager responsible for the overall outcome. This mindset kept me from feeling powerless even during a frightening time."

The Healthcare Hacker's Toolkit™

Effective health CEOs develop specific tools and techniques for navigating the system's complexity. The following toolkit components build on the knowledge you've gained in previous chapters:

1. **Your complete, organized health records** (as discussed in Chapter 4) form the foundation of your healthcare strategy. These records provide the data you need to identify patterns, prevent redundant testing, and ensure all providers have complete information.

2. **A care coordination system** that works for your personal style and needs. This might be a physical binder, a digital spreadsheet, a specialized app, or a combination of tools. The specific format matters less than having a system that helps you track appointments, medications, symptoms, questions, and follow up items.

3. **A health narrative document** that concisely summarizes your health history, current conditions, medications, allergies, and concerns. This one or two page summary, updated regularly, becomes your "executive brief" that you share with new healthcare professionals to ensure they quickly grasp your complete health context.

4. **A provider evaluation rubric** that helps you systematically assess whether healthcare providers meet your standards for technical expertise, communication quality, respect for your time, and collaboration willingness.

5. **A network of information sources** beyond your immediate doctors, including reputable healthcare websites, patient communities, and healthcare quality resources that help you evaluate treatment options and doctor recommendations.

6. **A financial tracking system** that monitors healthcare expenses, insurance reimbursements, and billing discrepancies, allowing you to identify errors and unnecessary costs (building on the financial insights from Chapter 5).

These toolkit components provide the infrastructure for implementing specific healthcare management strategies. The most successful healthcare hackers customize these tools to fit their personal needs, health conditions, and communication styles.

This may seem overwhelming, however you can download additional resources at **unfaircare.com/resources** to help make assembling and customizing your own toolkit easy.

Healthcare Optimization: Empower Your Care Journey

Navigating healthcare today requires more than showing up to appointments and hoping for the best. It demands strategic participation, collaboration, and proactive management. By optimizing appointments, strengthening your care team, and defending your financial well-being, you can transform your healthcare experience from reactive to empowered.

In this guide, you will walk through three pivotal strategies that place you firmly in control, all while recognizing the realities patients face and offering practical steps you can start using today.

1. Mastering Appointment Optimization

Appointments are often rushed, leaving critical information undiscussed. However, a few key strategies can dramatically increase the value you get from every visit.

Before Your Appointment

- **Set an agenda:** Write down your top concerns, questions, and goals. Prioritize what must be addressed.
- **Gather information:** Track symptoms, medication responses, and any changes since your last visit. Bring recent test results if available.
- **Prepare a concise summary:** Be ready to give a quick, focused overview of your situation.
- **Research your condition:** A little self-education can lead to sharper, more productive conversations.
- **Send information early:** Many patients now email their agendas or notes to clinics 24-48 hours before their appointment. This small step can vastly improve dialogue and decision-making.

Michael, who manages several chronic conditions, emails a bullet-point agenda before every visit. "It gives my doctor time to think through my issues in advance," he says, "and our appointments have become way more productive as a result."

When Scheduling Appointments

- Book **first appointments of the day** to minimize delays.
- Aim for **midweek** appointments to allow time for follow-up before weekends.
- For chronic conditions, consider **quarterly check-ins** rather than annual visits.
- Coordinate medical and dental care to **integrate treatment plans** and improve outcomes.

Strengthen the Documentation Partnership

Your health record shapes future care decisions. It's crucial you have input, so take the following steps:

- Review previous notes for accuracy before each visit.
- Offer written symptom summaries for complex histories.
- Request visit notes promptly and correct any errors quickly.

Building this partnership shows your engagement. Most doctors will appreciate your collaboration once they realize it elevates the quality of your care.

2. Building a Collaborative Care Team

You deserve a care team that listens, collaborates, and empowers you. With a few smart approaches, you can shift from a passive patient role to a confident partner in decision-making.

⚖️ **Make Smarter Treatment Decisions**

Use the **Three Essential Questions** whenever treatment is proposed:

1. **What are all of my options?** (Including doing nothing or waiting.)

2. **What are the benefits** and **risks of each option?**

3. **Given my situation and values, what would you recommend and why?**

This approach transforms one-sided conversations into meaningful, collaborative planning.

Conduct Independent Research

While your doctor's advice is crucial, complement it with your own research:

- Consult **multiple reputable sources**, not just the first website you find.
- Look for studies with **large sample sizes and reproducible results**.
- Be wary of conflicts of interest (e.g., studies funded by industry).

When you bring well-sourced questions and insights to the table, you become a true partner in your care without undermining professional expertise.

Document Major Decisions

Keep a simple but thorough log of:

- The condition(s) being treated
- All treatment options considered
- Risks, benefits, and your rationale for the final choice
- Follow-up plan
- Success criteria

Clear documentation protects your future care, and ensures all your providers are on the same page.

3. Defending Your Financial and Health Interests

As you have previously learned, healthcare is riddled with hidden costs, communication bottlenecks, and segmented information. Protecting yourself means taking the lead in communication and financial defense.

Open Better Communication Channels

Traditional healthcare communication is slow and convoluted. Build faster, clearer access by:

- Establishing emergency protocols (know how to reach your doctor directly).
- Negotiating secure direct messaging access for non-urgent issues.
- Building relationships with key staff members who can expedite help when needed.

You aren't asking for "special treatment". You're setting up appropriate, efficient ways to keep your health on track.

Use Prepared Communication

When you reach out to anyone on your healthcare team:

- Start with a **clear goal** ("I need a medication refill" vs. "I have some questions...")
- Be **brief and focused** with necessary context.
- Highlight specific questions and suggest response timelines.

Efficient communication respects your provider's time, and dramatically improves how quickly you get the answers you need.

Facilitate Provider Coordination

When your healthcare professionals don't talk to each other, critical information falls through the cracks. Step in:

- Actively request, collect, and share medical and dental records yourself.
- Create summary sheets that highlight essential details for each doctor.

- Schedule strategic appointments, so one specialist's findings can inform the next.

This kind of proactive coordination prevents gaps that could otherwise lead to delays, errors, or unnecessary costs.

The Quantified Self

Healthcare hackers increasingly use self-tracking tools to monitor health metrics and identify potential issues before they become symptomatic. Effective approaches include:

- **Establishing personal baselines** for key health indicators like blood pressure, resting heart rate, weight, energy levels, and mood
- **Tracking trends over time** rather than focusing on absolute values
- **Correlating changes with lifestyle factors** like diet, exercise, stress, or sleep
- **Sharing relevant tracking data with professionals** in organized, meaningful formats
- **Using wearable devices and apps** to automate data collection where appropriate

This quantified approach transforms vague awareness into actionable information that can guide both prevention and early intervention strategies.

Mary, who has a family history of heart disease, developed a sophisticated tracking system: "I monitor my blood pressure, resting heart rate, sleep quality, and activity levels daily, plus track key blood markers quarterly. This data has helped me identify how specific foods, activities, and stressors affect my cardiovascular health. When I noticed subtle trending changes in my metrics, I was able to adjust my exercise and stress management routines before problems developed."

The Emergency Dossier™

Create compact, accessible emergency dossiers containing essential information for crisis care. These typically include:

- Critical medical and dental conditions
- Allergies
- Current medications with dosages
- Emergency contacts and healthcare proxy information
- Primary care and specialist provider details
- Recent relevant test results
- Advance directive summary
- Insurance information

These dossiers can exist as printed cards, within smartphone apps, cloud documents, USB drives, and often in multiple formats to ensure accessibility in different scenarios.

Stacy, who travels frequently for work, found herself prepared when a dental emergency struck. "I was giving a presentation in Phoenix when my crown came loose. I immediately used the Cair app on my phone to connect with my dentist back home through teledentistry. She assessed the situation visually and accessed my dental records right from the app. She then shared my complete treatment history and X-rays with a local dentist she recommended through Cair's secure record sharing system. When I arrived at the office an hour later, the dentist had already reviewed my records, including my previous treatment notes. They had the exact specifications for my crown and completed the reattachment efficiently. What could have been a multiday ordeal that derailed my business trip was resolved in a couple of hours. I now keep all my dental information updated in Cair. It has been invaluable for both routine care and emergencies, no matter where I am."

Advance Advocacy

It is important to establish systems to ensure effective advocacy during health crises when you might be unable to advocate for yourself. These systems typically include:

- **Designated healthcare proxies** with detailed understanding of your values and preferences
- **Written advance directives** addressing both end-of-life and nonterminal care preferences
- **Emergency provider lists** identifying both preferred and nonpreferred hospitals and specialists
- **Family access to records** through appropriate HIPAA authorizations and sharing with key providers

These systems provide support during vulnerable periods when healthcare quality depends heavily on effective representation of your interests.

Final Thought: Healthcare Is a Team Sport. And You Are the Captain.

By preparing strategically, collaborating confidently, and defending your interests wisely, you can create a healthcare experience that's safer, smarter, and more satisfying. You don't need a medical degree to play an active role in your care. Just a clear plan, the right tools, and the willingness to engage.

You are not just a patient. You are the leader of your healthcare.

Action Items

Before you learn how to build your personal care team in detail in the next chapter, consider taking these immediate steps to begin hacking better care:

1. **Schedule a prevention focused appointment** with your primary care doctor specifically to discuss a comprehensive prevention strategy rather than addressing immediate concerns.

2. **Create your Emergency Dossier**™ containing essential information and data for crisis situations, and ensure key people know how to access it.

These steps establish the foundation for a more sophisticated approach to healthcare navigation. One that acknowledges system realities while refusing to be limited by them. For help aggregating this information, go to **unfaircare.com/resources**.

Healthcare hacking isn't about circumventing appropriate care or rejecting doctor expertise. Rather, it's about creating systems and approaches that enhance the care you receive by compensating for structural limitations baked into our healthcare models.

The healthcare system may be dysfunctional, but your approach to it doesn't have to be.

Become the CEO of your health. Take command of your care.

PART III

Designing Your Care Model

SEVEN

Build Your Personal Care Team

"None of us is as smart as all of us." —Ken Blanchard

David had always prided himself on his self-reliance. At 52, he managed his health the same way he approached his business, handling issues individually as they arose, seeing specialists when necessary, and moving on. This approach seemed efficient until a constellation of seemingly unrelated symptoms began affecting his quality of life.

Over eighteen months, David consulted seven different specialists: a gastroenterologist for digestive issues, a neurologist for headaches, a rheumatologist for joint pain, a sleep specialist for insomnia, a cardiologist for palpitations, a dermatologist for rashes, and a psychiatrist for anxiety. Each specialist ordered tests within their domain, prescribed medications for specific symptoms, and suggested follow up appointments.

Yet despite this parade of expertise and a growing medication list, David's overall health deteriorated. The breaking point came when his pharmacist called about a potentially dangerous interaction between medications prescribed by different specialists, neither of whom knew about the other's treatment plan.

"That was my wake up call," David later explained. "I realized I didn't have seven different health problems. I had one body experiencing multiple symptoms, and nobody was connecting the dots."

With this insight, David completely reorganized his approach to healthcare. He found a primary care physician specializing in complex cases and gave her copies of all his specialist records. Together, they identified patterns suggesting an autoimmune condition exacerbated by stress and poor sleep. They created a collaborative treatment plan and assembled a coordinated team of professionals who communicated regularly.

Within six months, David was taking fewer medications and experiencing significant improvement in his symptoms. As importantly, he no longer felt like he was navigating a confusing medical maze alone.

"The difference wasn't just better treatment, it was having a team approach where everyone communicated and worked together," David reflected. "For the first time, I felt like I had healthcare partners rather than just providers."

David's experience illustrates why building a personal care team, rather than simply collecting individual healthcare providers, represents a crucial strategy for getting the care you deserve. In this chapter, you will explore how to identify, evaluate, select, and organize the right healthcare professionals to create your optimal care team.

Why Teams Outperform Individuals

Healthcare has traditionally operated on a model of individual expertise. Expertise such as the brilliant diagnostician, the skilled surgeon, and the experienced specialist. While individual excellence certainly matters, research consistently shows that well coordinated teams deliver superior outcomes compared to collections of individuals, no matter how capable those individuals may be.

This team advantage emerges from several factors:

Complementary Knowledge and Perspectives

No single healthcare professional, regardless of training or brilliance, possesses comprehensive expertise across all health domains. A cardiologist might miss the oral health connection to heart disease discussed in Chapter 2. A dentist might not recognize how a medication prescribed by a rheumatologist affects dental treatment. A primary care physician might overlook subtle nutritional factors a registered dietitian would immediately identify.

In short, teams with diverse expertise create a collective intelligence that exceeds any individual contribution. They see patterns and connections that specialists focused on single systems might miss. They challenge each other's assumptions and blind spots, leading to more accurate diagnoses and comprehensive treatment plans.

Consider Teresa's experience with chronic migraines. After years of neurologist prescribed medications providing minimal relief, she assembled a team including her neurologist, a physical therapist specializing in cervical spine issues, a dentist with temporomandibular joint expertise, and a nutritionist familiar with food trigger patterns. This integrated approach revealed multiple contributing factors, including jaw misalignment, cervical tension, and specific food sensitivities, that no single doctor had fully identified. Addressing these factors in coordination reduced her migraine frequency by over 70%.

Reduced Cognitive Bias

Individual healthcare professionals, despite their training, remain susceptible to cognitive biases that can compromise care quality, including:

- **Confirmation bias**: Seeking information that confirms initial impressions while overlooking contradictory evidence
- **Availability bias**: Overestimating the likelihood of diagnoses they've recently encountered
- **Anchoring bias**: Placing too much weight on first information received and failing to adjust sufficiently
- **Diagnosis momentum**: Accepting previous diagnoses without sufficient reconsideration

Teams naturally mitigate these biases through collective evaluation and different perspectives. When multiple care providers review the same information, they're more likely to identify alternative explanations, question assumptions, and catch potential errors before they affect treatment.

Continuity Across Episodes

Healthcare often splinters across acute episodes, with little connectivity between events. Teams provide continuity that individual doctors cannot, particularly when the team members include both episodic specialists (like surgeons) and longitudinal providers (like primary care physicians).

This continuity proves especially valuable during transitions, from hospital to home, from one treatment approach to another, or from one life stage to the next. Team members who maintain ongoing relationships with you can preserve crucial context that would otherwise be lost during these transitions.

🤝 No One Can Outperform a Well-Aligned Team

Brilliance matters.

But alignment multiplies it.

When individuals operate in silos, their talents compete.

When teams operate in sync, their talents compound.

Healthcare is too complex, too fast-moving, and too high-stakes for solo heroics.

Teams win. Not because they're perfect, but because they catch each other's blind spots.

Precision, creativity, and accountability are team sports.

The Architecture of an Effective Care Team

An optimal personal care team isn't simply a random collection of doctors. It has intentional structure, clear roles, and defined communication patterns. While specific team composition varies based on individual health needs, most effective care teams share common architectural elements.

Doctor Selection

The healthcare professionals you choose dramatically influence your healthcare experience. Unfortunately, the traditional system often treats doctor selection as an afterthought, assigning patients based on insurance networks and availability rather than quality or compatibility.

Effective healthcare hackers develop sophisticated approaches to identifying and selecting optimal clinicians.

Beyond Insurance Directories

Insurance provider directories offer limited information, typically just basic credentials, location, and contact information. To manage provider selection effectively, supplement these directories with:

- **Quality ratings from independent organizations** like Leapfrog Group (for hospitals), Healthgrades, or specialty specific quality initiatives
- **Board certification verification** through the American Board of Medical Specialties, your state's Board of Dentistry or specialty board websites
- **Disciplinary action checks** through your state's medical or dental board
- **Practice research** using sites like ProPublica's "Dollars for Docs" that reveal financial relationships between providers and pharmaceutical companies

- **Patient reviews** from reputable sources, focusing less on personality assessments and more on your focused aspects of care experience

Alexandra, who relocated frequently for work, developed a systematic approach, "Before selecting new doctors in each city, I create a spreadsheet of candidates who meet my basic criteria. These include board certification, hospital affiliations, and insurance participation. Then I research each one's communication style, scope of practice, and patient feedback. This process takes time upfront, but has consistently led me to exceptional providers."

The Interview Approach

Most patients simply accept the first available appointment with an in-network provider. In contrast, healthcare hackers approach initial visits as mutual interviews, using the opportunity to evaluate whether the doctor meets their standards while also giving the clinician a chance to determine whether they can effectively address the patient's needs.

An effective provider interview involves preparing specific questions related to your health concerns, carefully observing how the clinician communicates, noting whether they interrupt, how they respond to questions, and how clearly they explain complex topics. It also includes gauging the clinician's openness to collaboration by expressing your desire to be actively involved in care decisions.

Beyond clinical and communication assessment, it's important to evaluate logistical aspects of care, such as appointment availability, response times to questions, and how well the practice coordinates with other professionals.

Discussing the doctor's general philosophy, particularly their views on prevention, lifestyle factors, and preferred treatment approaches, can offer insight into whether their approach aligns with your values.

Many proactive patients even schedule brief "meet and greet" appointments solely for the purpose of this interview, separating the process of provider selection from any immediate health needs. While insurance often doesn't cover these visits, the upfront investment can yield substantial long-term benefits in care quality and satisfaction.

Building Your Care Team Strategically

Beyond selecting individual doctors, people engaged in their healthcare can construct integrated care teams designed around their specific needs. This strategic team-building includes:

- **Identifying a primary coordinator,** typically a primary care physician or sometimes a trusted specialist for patients with dominant chronic conditions, who serves as the hub of your care network

- **Selecting specialists who communicate effectively** with your primary doctor and with each other

- **Choosing allied health professionals** like physical therapists, chiropractors, nutritionists, mental health professionals, or health coaches who address dimensions of health beyond traditional medical care

- **Considering complementary providers** like acupuncturists, massage therapists, or functional medicine practitioners when appropriate for your health needs

- **Incorporating all your dental professionals**, including a primary dentist that you can coordinate into your overall health team, recognizing the crucial oral-systemic connections discussed in Chapters 2 and 3

Recognize that optimal teams vary based on individual health needs. Someone managing diabetes might assemble an endocrinologist, nutritionist, ophthalmologist, podiatrist, and periodontist (given the diabetes-periodontal disease connection). Someone with autoimmune issues might focus on rheumatology, gastroenterology, and functional medicine.

The key is intentionally constructing your team rather than accumulating random providers through referrals alone.

The Primary Coordinator Role

Every effective healthcare team needs a coordinator, someone who maintains a comprehensive view of your health and ensures seamless communication among specialists. This role can be filled by different types of providers, depending on your individual needs.

It might be a primary care physician with a holistic approach and strong communication skills, or an internist who specializes in managing complex, multi system conditions. Some patients find this coordination within a "medical home" practice, which is specifically structured to streamline care across multiple clinicians.

For older adults with multiple health issues, a geriatrician often takes the lead. In certain cases, the specialist managing your primary health concern, such as an oncologist for cancer patients or a rheumatologist for autoimmune disorders, naturally steps into the coordinating role.

Regardless of who fills the position, this provider functions as your healthcare "general contractor," overseeing a team of specialists like subcontractors. Their job is to focus on your overall health, not just isolated symptoms or systems. They help interpret specialist recommendations, resolve potential conflicts in treatment plans, and ensure that no critical aspect of your well-being is lost in the shuffle of siloed care.

While your primary care coordinator acts as the "quarterback" of your team remember, as you learned in Chapter 6, you are the captain.

Dr. Martin, a primary care physician who frequently serves as a coordinator, describes his approach: "I see myself as the patient's chief medical officer. My job isn't to know everything about every condition, it's to know which specialists to involve, when to challenge their recommendations, how to integrate different perspectives, and most importantly, how to translate everything into a cohesive plan that makes sense for the patient's life."

The Specialist Constellation

Once you've established a primary care coordinator, the next step is to build a team of specialists tailored to your specific health needs. These may include disease-specific experts such as cardiologists, endocrinologists, or oncologists, as well as system-focused specialists like gastroenterologists or neurologists who address particular body systems.

For surgical or interventional needs, procedural specialists play a key role, while rehabilitation specialists such as physical and occupational therapists help support recovery and long-term function. Mental health professionals, including psychiatrists, psychologists, and counselors, also serve as essential team members when emotional or cognitive support is needed.

Remember, effective specialist selection requires more than just clinical expertise. It's equally important to choose doctors who are willing to collaborate as part of a larger care team rather than operate as isolated experts. Specialists differ not only in their medical approaches but also in their practice models. Some focus narrowly on procedures, while others adopt a more comprehensive view of their specialty.

Choosing the right fit means selecting specialists whose style and philosophy align with your personal preferences and long-term care goals.

The Dental Integration Component

Any comprehensive care team must include oral health expertise. When adding dental professionals to your healthcare team, look specifically for those who understand systemic health connections and communicate effectively with medical counterparts.

This includes selecting a primary dentist who understands and actively considers the links between oral conditions and systemic diseases, as well as dental specialists, such as periodontists, endodontists, or oral surgeons, when their expertise is required. Equally important are the communication channels established between dental and medical doctors, ensuring that care remains coordinated and comprehensive.

The most effective dental team members recognize that their responsibility extends beyond oral health. They are attuned to systemic conditions, like diabetes, that influence dental treatment plans, carefully consider potential medication interactions, and proactively reach out to medical colleagues when oral findings may signal broader health concerns.

Not Just a Dentist. A Health Ally

Most dentists still operate in silos. But the best ones see the full picture.

Look for dental professionals who understand how oral health connects to conditions like diabetes and heart disease and communicate clearly across disciplines to keep your care connected.

Your mouth isn't separate from your body.

Your dental care shouldn't be either.

The Lifestyle and Prevention Element

Conventional medical teams often concentrate on diagnosing and treating disease, rather than fostering the creation of health. In contrast, truly comprehensive care teams expand beyond this reactive model to include professionals who specialize in lifestyle medicine, prevention, and health optimization.

These include registered dietitians who offer evidence-based nutritional guidance tailored to individual needs, as well as exercise physiologists or physical therapists who design appropriate physical activity plans to support strength, mobility, and cardiovascular health.

Health coaches play a crucial role in facilitating sustainable behavior change, while sleep specialists help address a vital but frequently overlooked pillar of health.

Additionally, stress management experts contribute tools and techniques that support psychological resilience and emotional wellbeing. These professionals focus on foundational aspects of health that are often underemphasized in traditional medical settings, despite their significant influence on disease risk, treatment effectiveness, and overall quality of life.

Betty, who reversed her pre-diabetes through lifestyle interventions, credits her expanded care team: "My endocrinologist identified the problem and prescribed medication, but it was my dietitian, health coach, and exercise physiologist who actually solved it. Working together, they helped me make sustainable changes that no single professional could have. Two years later, my blood sugar is normal, and without any medication."

Complementary Care Integration

Many patients find significant value in including carefully selected complementary providers as part of their care teams. These may include acupuncturists for pain management and targeted conditions, chiropractors for musculoskeletal issues, and massage therapists who support both specific therapeutic goals and general wellbeing.

Mind-body practitioners, such as those teaching meditation, yoga, or other mindfulness-based techniques, can be instrumental in managing stress and enhancing emotional health.

Many patients may find benefit in working with functional medicine providers, who focus on uncovering root causes and addressing biochemical individuality, and often bring a personalized, systems-based perspective to chronic or complex health challenges.

The key to integrating complementary care effectively lies in choosing professionals who are collaborative, understand the appropriate limits of their practice, communicate clearly with the broader team, and respect your role in guiding your treatment choices.

When thoughtfully incorporated, these practitioners can address dimensions of health that conventional medicine may manage less effectively, especially in areas such as chronic pain, stress-related conditions, and functional disorders.

Looking Beyond Credentials

Conventional wisdom suggests choosing healthcare providers based primarily on credentials, institutional affiliations, and experience. While credentials and experience still matter, research increasingly shows that factors like communication, collaboration, and patient-centeredness are stronger predictors of care quality and team effectiveness.

Practice System Alignment

A doctor's practice structure plays a crucial role in determining how effectively they can function as part of your care team. It's important to consider whether their systems support or obstruct collaboration.

Key indicators include the use of electronic health records that allow for secure information sharing, clearly defined communication protocols for working with other clinicians, and scheduling flexibility to accommodate urgent issues or joint appointments.

The presence of a support team that can assist with record management and coordination of tasks, along with prompt response times to questions and follow-up needs, also signals a well-integrated practice.

Ultimately, a healthcare professional who operates within a system designed to promote teamwork will contribute far more effectively to your overall care than one who must constantly battle operational barriers, regardless of how well-intentioned they may be.

Philosophical Compatibility

Healthcare providers operate within a wide range of philosophical frameworks that shape their approach to everything from diagnosis to treatment recommendations. These differences aren't simply a matter of right versus wrong; they reflect legitimate variations in clinical perspective and professional orientation. Ideally, you should align your personal values and preferences with that of every professional you see.

While this may not be entirely possible, when assembling your care team, consider whether potential doctors share your views on key issues that are important to you. These can include intervention thresholds, whether they prefer to treat proactively or take a watch-and-wait approach, and their orientation toward pharmaceuticals, whether they see medication as a first-line solution or a last resort.

Also important are their attitudes toward patient autonomy, ranging from directive styles to collaborative decision-making, and how they define valid evidence, favoring traditional research or being open to emerging approaches.

While your team doesn't need to consist of philosophical clones, some baseline alignment is essential. Diverse perspectives can enrich your care, but fundamental conflicts in philosophy may lead to friction that compromises coordination and effectiveness.

Facilitating Team Functionality

Even the most carefully selected healthcare team requires active coordination to function effectively. As your healthcare CEO (as discussed in Chapter 6), you play a crucial role in facilitating your team's operation.

The Health Central Information Hub

Effective teams need shared information. Since healthcare lacks comprehensive information sharing infrastructure, create your own central information repository, as part of your toolkit, that includes:

- **Complete health records** from all providers (as outlined in Chapter 4)
- **Current medication lists** with dosages and prescribing providers
- **Recent test results** in chronological order
- **Treatment plans** from each team member
- **Your goals and preferences** for various aspects of care, as detailed above in this chapter

This hub might exist as a physical binder, a digital folder system, a secure cloud based platform, or a specialized health record app. The specific format matters less than having a system that allows you to share consistent, comprehensive information with all team members.

HEALTH DATA HUB

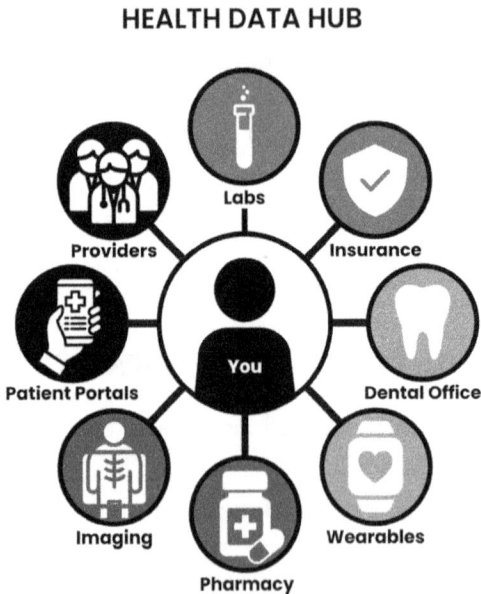

The Communication Matrix

Developing a structured approach to team communication is essential for coordinated care. This includes clarifying who needs to receive what information from which providers, identifying each team member's preferred communication methods, and establishing expected response timeframes for different types of communication, whether routine updates or urgent concerns.

It's also important to define documentation standards for shared information to ensure clarity and consistency, along with a clear process for escalating coordination needs when time is critical.

Many proactive patients take this a step further by creating communication matrices, simple tables that map out which providers should receive specific types of information from others. These matrices place the patient at the center, defining their role as the primary connection point among team members and making care coordination more intentional and effective.

Michael, who manages a complex cardiac condition, developed a color-coded system: "I created a simple chart showing which doctors need what information from others. Green means 'always share,' yellow means 'share significant changes,' and red means 'urgent notification required.' This clarity prevents both communication gaps and information overload."

The Regular Review Process

Effective care teams require ongoing evaluation and periodic adjustment to stay aligned with your evolving health needs. Establishing a regular review process, ideally at least quarterly, can help ensure that care remains well-coordinated.

This includes updating all providers on significant developments reported by other team members, identifying any emerging conflicts in treatment recommendations, and reassessing whether each clinician continues to contribute meaningful value.

As your condition or goals change, team composition may also need to evolve. This review process can take several forms: formal team meetings, which are increasingly feasible through telehealth; sequential appointments arranged to encourage cross-communication; or even your own systematic check-in, followed by personalized updates shared with each provider.

Whatever the method, consistent reflection and adjustment are key to maintaining a high-functioning, responsive care team.

When Team Members Don't Meet Expectations

Even carefully selected healthcare teams sometimes include providers who don't function effectively within the team structure. When a provider isn't meeting your team's expectations, it is best to leverage direct, respectful communication.

Start off by clearly identifying the specific issue, whether it's poor communication, conflicting recommendations, or lack of follow-through, and explain your expectations for team-based care. Be explicit about the changes you'd like to see in their participation and document the conversation along with any commitments they make.

It's also helpful to agree on a timeline for reassessing progress. Many providers respond positively to this level of clarity, especially when they understand how their role contributes to your broader, coordinated care strategy.

If a direct conversation doesn't lead to improved team function, consider implementing more structured methods of integration. One approach is to schedule three-way appointments that include both the challenging provider and your primary coordinator to align expectations and promote collaboration.

You might also introduce standardized communication templates (as you will find at **unfaircare.com/resources**) to streamline information sharing or establish regular check-ins focused specifically on team integration.

Additionally, offering positive reinforcement when the professional demonstrates team-oriented behavior can encourage ongoing engagement. These strategies often help well-intentioned professionals move beyond ingrained habits that may be unintentionally hindering effective teamwork.

The Replacement Decision

When a provider consistently shows an inability or unwillingness to function as an effective team member, despite clear expectations and structured support, it is likely time to consider a replacement.

Begin by documenting the specific ways the provider has failed to meet the team's coordination requirements. From there, identify potential replacements who demonstrate a stronger orientation toward collaborative care.

As you manage the transition, prioritize continuity by ensuring that records are transferred smoothly and responsibilities are clearly reassigned. Communicate your reasons for the change with professionalism and clarity, both to the outgoing provider and to the remaining team.

Finally, reflect on whether this experience highlights any adjustments needed in your team selection or evaluation process. Although replacing a clinician requires short-term effort, continuing to tolerate ineffective participation can compromise your entire care structure, leading to greater workload, confusion, and poorer outcomes over time.

Financial Considerations in Team Building

Healthcare teams operate within financial constraints that require careful navigation. Building on the financial insights introduced in Chapter 5, patients can design sustainable care teams by combining different approaches based on coverage, value, and your direct investment in your care. The following are different, equally effective, approaches to building your team, based on your personal financial considerations:

The Strategic Insurance Approach

The strategic insurance approach to designing your care teams involves working within insurance networks to manage costs effectively. This means selecting in-network providers for roles that involve frequent visits or high utilization, while preserving out-of-network flexibility for specialized or high-impact needs.

Fully utilizing preventive services covered by insurance and leveraging "medical necessity" provisions can help justify coordination efforts. When coverage is denied, presenting appeals framed with team-based rationales can sometimes lead to successful reconsideration.

Many healthcare hackers use this model to stretch their healthcare dollars, relying on insurance for some team members while choosing to pay out of pocket for others whose value justifies the additional investment.

The Value-based Approach

Another tactic is the value-based selection method, which evaluates clinicians through a more nuanced lens than just their price tag. This approach considers a provider's total cost impact, outcome effectiveness relative to expense, time efficiency in addressing health concerns, and their contributions to coordinated care that helps avoid duplication or disconnection.

This approach also emphasizes prevention as a cost-saving strategy over the long term. Patients using this model understand that the cheapest option is not always the best. In fact, in many cases, professionals who charge more deliver better overall value when viewed through the lens of health outcomes or reduced long-term spending.

The Direct Payment Approach

Finally, the direct payment option can be especially effective for certain roles on the care team, or if you would like to seek the best care possible, regardless of the cost. Paying providers directly and bypassing the constraints of insurance, can oftentimes create better alignment between patient and doctor, especially in roles that require deep, ongoing engagement.

Many times this works best when working with primary coordinators who provide comprehensive oversight, preventive specialists not well supported by insurance plans, integrative providers who focus on root causes, and health coaches who help sustain behavior change.

Be aware that some clinics may offer significant discounts for direct-pay arrangements, so even if the cost of your care is not your primary concern, it still makes sense to seek open, transparent pricing from your directly-paid providers.

Also, while this method requires more upfront investment, it often yields greater value through patient-centered relationships that are not compromised by third-party incentives or restrictions.

Action Items

As you develop prevention strategies more deeply in the next chapter, consider taking these immediate actions to begin building your personal care team:

1. **Evaluate your current healthcare relationships** using the team-oriented criteria discussed in this chapter. Identify which existing providers demonstrate strong team qualities and which may need replacement or supplementation.

2. **Create your communication matrix** identifying which professionals need to share what information with each other, with yourself as the central connection point.

Again, to make this process easier, check out **unfaircare.com /resources**.

These steps begin transforming your healthcare experience from a collection of separated provider relationships into a coordinated team focused on your comprehensive health needs. This transformation doesn't happen overnight, but even modest progress toward team-based care yields significant benefits in treatment coordination, outcome improvement, and reduced overall healthcare costs.

Your health deserves nothing less than the collective wisdom, diverse expertise, and coordinated effort that only a true healthcare team can provide.

Stop waiting for a better healthcare team to magically form around you. Assemble it. Identify your key professionals, including primary care, dentist, and specialists. Then demand cross-communication.

Map out your care team like your life depends on it. Because it does.

EIGHT

Prevent First, Treat Smarter

"An ounce of prevention is worth a pound of cure."
—Benjamin Franklin, whose wisdom on
health preceded modern medicine

Elena had always considered herself healthy. At 41, she exercised regularly, maintained a reasonable weight, and had no obvious health complaints beyond occasional stress and fatigue that she attributed to her demanding career and family life. Her annual physical examinations typically concluded with her physician saying, "Everything looks normal," followed by a quick handshake and a reminder to schedule next year's visit.

When a corporate wellness program offered comprehensive preventive screening, Elena participated primarily to receive the insurance discount. The results shocked her; borderline blood pressure, pre-diabetic glucose levels, significant vitamin D deficiency, and early stage periodontal disease. None of these conditions had triggered sufficient symptoms to prompt concern, yet collectively they placed her on a trajectory toward serious health problems.

"I was stunned," Elena recalled. "I'd been seeing doctors and dentists regularly for years. How could so many issues be developing without anyone raising alarm bells?"

The answer lay in the fundamental orientation of her healthcare. Reactive rather than proactive, focused on diagnosing obvious disease rather than optimizing health and preventing future problems. Her doctors weren't negligent; they were simply practicing within a system designed to address problems after they develop rather than prevent them from occurring.

Elena's wake up call prompted a complete reorientation of her approach to healthcare. Working with a prevention focused primary care physician and the team she assembled using principles from the previous chapter, she developed a comprehensive prevention strategy addressing multiple dimensions of health. This included more sophisticated cardiometabolic monitoring, a personalized nutrition plan, stress management techniques, improved sleep habits, and enhanced dental care targeting her periodontal issues.

Two years later, all her biomarkers had improved significantly. Her periodontal disease had reversed, her blood pressure normalized, her glucose levels improved, and her energy increased dramatically. Perhaps most importantly, her relationship with healthcare transformed from being a passive receipt of episodic "checkups" to her active engagement in ongoing health optimization.

"I used to think being healthy meant not being sick," Elena reflected. "Now I understand that true health is proactive, not just the absence of disease. The difference in how I feel is remarkable, and I've likely avoided serious problems that were developing silently."

Elena's experience illustrates the powerful potential of prevention oriented healthcare. An approach that remains underemphasized in our treatment focused system. In this chapter, you will learn specific strategies for reorienting your healthcare toward prevention, early intervention, and optimal wellness rather than merely responding to established disease.

The Prevention Paradox Revisited

As introduced in Chapter 1, our healthcare system demonstrates a fundamental paradox: while prevention offers the greatest potential for improving health outcomes and reducing costs, the system allocates minimal resources to preventive approaches and creates structural barriers to their implementation.

This systemic failure has profound implications for individuals navigating healthcare. Unfortunately, you will rarely receive comprehensive preventive care unless you actively initiate, coordinate, and sometimes even design it yourself.

Understanding the dimensions of this prevention paradox helps explain why traditional healthcare often fails to deliver appropriate preventive services even when clinicians have good intentions.

The Reimbursement Reality

The unfortunate payment structure we examined earlier manifests clearly in preventive care. Knowing this economic reality allows you to adapt your approach and ensure prevention receives appropriate priority despite financial disincentives.

For example, a 30-minute discussion about evidence-based lifestyle modifications that might prevent diabetes generates a fraction of the revenue of procedures treating diabetes complications.

This financial disincentive shapes clinical practice patterns even among doctors who intellectually recognize prevention's importance. Faced with packed schedules and financial pressures, clinicians naturally gravitate toward billable procedures rather than time consuming preventive counseling.

The average primary care appointment lasts less than 18 minutes, barely enough time to address acute concerns, let alone develop comprehensive prevention strategies (Chen et al. 2009). Meaningful preventive care requires thorough assessment, personalized planning, education, and follow up, elements that simply cannot fit into hurried appointments.

This time compression affects both the quantity and quality of preventive services. Clinicians may technically "check the box" for preventive requirements without providing the thorough approaches actually needed for effective prevention.

The Reactive Mindset

Perhaps most fundamentally, conventional healthcare operates from a reactive rather than proactive orientation. The system intervenes primarily when symptoms appear or screening detects significant problems. This orientation permeates everything from appointment scheduling to diagnostic protocols to treatment planning.

Even traditional "preventive" services often actually represent early detection rather than true prevention, identifying diseases in early stages rather than preventing their development. While early detection certainly improves outcomes compared to late diagnosis, it represents a limited form of prevention focused on disease rather than health.

🔥 We Wait for the Fire, Then Look for a Hose

Imagine if firefighters only responded once a house was engulfed in flames, and called it "prevention" because they arrived before it collapsed.

That's how much of healthcare still works today.

We don't invest deeply in true prevention, like addressing diet, stress, oral health, environment, and early lifestyle triggers.

Instead, we catch diseases just early enough to manage them, often too late to avoid them. It's not just inefficient. It's expensive, traumatic, and avoidable.

Health isn't the absence of disease. It's the presence of resilience. And resilience requires foresight, not damage control.

The Prevention Spectrum: Beyond Basic Screenings

Moving beyond the system's limitations requires understanding that prevention encompasses a much broader spectrum than the basic screenings and immunizations typically associated with common "preventive care." Comprehensive prevention includes multiple levels and dimensions, many of which receive minimal attention in conventional healthcare.

Primary Prevention Priority

Primary prevention, intervening before disease develops, offers the greatest potential for long-term health impact, yet it remains one of the most neglected areas in traditional healthcare. Truly effective primary prevention strategies go well beyond generic advice and focus on individualized, proactive interventions.

This includes optimizing nutrition based on personal metabolic needs and genetic factors, engaging in physical activity that matches current fitness levels and is sustainable over time. Also, adopting stress management techniques that mitigate the physiological effects of chronic stress should be incorporated into these preventive strategies.

Improving sleep quality is another essential element, given the foundational role sleep plays in overall health. Reducing exposure to environmental toxins, from pollutants and household chemicals to workplace hazards, further protects the body from preventable harm.

As we have discussed in previous chapters, oral health maintenance is equally critical, as preventing conditions like periodontal disease can reduce systemic inflammation and lower the risk of related health issues.

Unlike early disease detection or screening, these strategies address the actual root causes of illness. Yet, despite their profound potential, traditional medical systems often offer little more than surface-level advice such as "eat healthy and exercise," leaving patients without the depth of support needed to truly prevent disease.

Allen, a 45-year-old with a strong family history of heart disease, experienced this limitation firsthand: "My doctor told me to 'watch my diet' after seeing my family history, but offered no specific guidance. It wasn't until I worked with a preventive cardiologist and nutritionist that I learned about specific dietary patterns, supplements, and exercise protocols shown to significantly reduce cardiac risk. This detailed approach was entirely different from the vague recommendations I'd received for years."

Secondary Prevention

Secondary prevention, identifying and addressing conditions at their earliest and most treatable stages, is the most commonly practiced form of prevention in conventional healthcare, typically through standardized screening tests. However, this approach often suffers from serious limitations.

Screening protocols are frequently one-size-fits-all, failing to account for individual risk factors, personal history, or genetic predispositions. High-risk individuals may not be monitored often enough, while the limited scope of standard screenings can miss important health markers entirely.

Borderline results that fall short of a disease diagnosis often receive little or no follow-up, and screenings across different domains, such as physical, behavioral, or dental, are rarely well integrated.

To enhance the effectiveness of secondary prevention, more sophisticated approaches are needed. This involves getting screenings that are tailored to your personal health risks and family history, using more detailed lab tests to catch early signs of problems, aiming for the best possible health levels instead of just staying in the "normal" range, and keeping track of your results over time to spot issues before they get serious.

Tertiary Prevention

Tertiary prevention focuses on helping people live as well as possible when they already have health conditions. It aims to reduce complications and improve daily functioning, but traditional healthcare often doesn't go far enough in this area. An effective approach involves creating a full plan to manage every part of the condition, not just the most obvious symptoms.

It also means helping people build on what they can do, rather than only focusing on their limitations. Strategies should be tailored to prevent specific complications based on each person's unique risks, and support should go beyond just treating disease to improving overall quality of life.

As conditions and treatments change, care plans should be regularly reviewed and adjusted. This more complete approach moves chronic disease care from simply managing problems to helping people stay as healthy and capable as possible, even with ongoing conditions.

Robert, living with psoriatic arthritis for a decade, experienced this transformation: "For years, my care focused exclusively on immuno-suppressant medications to control joint inflammation. When I found a rheumatologist who approached tertiary prevention comprehensively, everything changed. We addressed my previously overlooked gum inflammation, sleep quality, specific exercise timing, stress management, and gut health. My medication needs decreased, my energy improved, and joint damage I'd been told was inevitable hasn't materialized."

Creating Your Personal Prevention Blueprint

Moving from conventional reactive care to comprehensive prevention requires developing your own prevention blueprint. A structured approach to promoting health rather than merely avoiding disease. While specific details vary based on individual needs, effective prevention blueprints share common elements:

Comprehensive Risk Assessment

Traditional risk assessment typically focuses on obvious factors like family history of major diseases, smoking status, and basic metrics like blood pressure and cholesterol. A truly comprehensive assessment expands to include:

- **Genetic predisposition analysis** through family history pattern recognition or formal genetic testing
- **Environmental exposure evaluation** of home, workplace, and community toxin sources
- **Behavioral pattern assessment** identifying habits that impact health trajectories
- **Psychosocial factor consideration** including stress patterns, social connections, and purpose
- **Oral health status** recognizing its connections to systemic health as explored in Chapter 2
- **Nutritional pattern analysis** beyond basic calorie and macronutrient intake
- **Movement and fitness evaluation** assessing both quantity and quality of physical activity
- **Sleep quality assessment** using both subjective and objective measures

This multidimensional risk assessment provides the foundation for truly personalized prevention strategies rather than generic recommendations. While conventional healthcare professionals rarely offer such comprehensive assessment, members of your healthcare team (as established in Chapter 7) can collectively contribute to this broader evaluation.

The Monitoring Matrix

To prevent health problems effectively, it's important to monitor different areas of your health in a clear and organized way. This means deciding which specific health markers to track based on your personal risks, how often each one should be checked, and what your ideal target ranges should be, not just what's considered "normal."

It also involves knowing which healthcare professionals or tools will handle each type of test, and making sure all the results are reviewed together to spot patterns that might otherwise be missed. By taking this structured approach, you turn random check-ups into a meaningful strategy that helps guide your long-term health and prevention goals.

Laura, with risk factors for multiple conditions, developed a sophisticated monitoring matrix: "I track 28 specific biomarkers at frequencies ranging from daily (like blood pressure) to annually (like comprehensive dental assessments). For each marker, I have three ranges: optimal, acceptable, and concerning. This system helps me identify subtle trends long before conventional medicine would detect a problem."

The Prevention Partnership Model

As with other aspects of care coordination we have already explored, prevention works best when you have a strong, collaborative relationship with healthcare professionals who support your proactive approach.

This kind of partnership involves clear communication about your health goals and preferences, along with shared decision-making when it comes to screenings and treatment options. It also means regularly reviewing your prevention plan to see what's working and what might need to change. Each professional plays a specific role based on their expertise and the way they approach care.

As part of the partnership, you should also stay informed about new research and prevention strategies that could benefit you. This model shifts the experience from one where the doctor makes all the decisions to one where you work together to shape a plan that fits your life and helps guide your long-term health.

Implementing Primary Prevention Strategies

While comprehensive prevention spans multiple levels, primary prevention, preventing disease development before it begins, offers the greatest potential impact on long term health. The following strategies help implement effective primary prevention beyond conventional healthcare's limited approaches:

The Nutritional Foundation

Nutrition is arguably the most powerful tool for primary prevention, yet it remains one of the most overlooked areas in conventional healthcare.

A truly effective nutritional approach goes far beyond the generic advice often given in standard medical settings. Rather it is adopting anti-inflammatory dietary patterns that are tailored to your unique metabolic needs, optimizing micronutrient levels to address common deficiencies that can have significant health effects, and using meal timing strategies that support metabolic function and cellular repair.

It also incorporates specific functional foods shown to help prevent the conditions you're personally at risk for, and customizing your nutritional plan based on how your body responds, rather than relying on one-size-fits-all recommendations. This more personalized, evidence-informed approach to nutrition stands in sharp contrast to the vague guidance most patients receive and plays a central role in building long-term health.

Thomas, with a family history of neurodegenerative disease, worked with a dietitian specializing in brain health: "We developed a specific protocol including omega-3 levels, antioxidant-rich foods, appropriate intermittent fasting, and targeted supplementation based on my genetic factors. This detailed approach went far beyond the generic guidance I'd previously received."

Movement Optimization

The prevention benefits of physical activity go far beyond just weight management, yet conventional healthcare rarely offers specific personalized guidance in this area. A comprehensive approach to movement includes a balanced mix of cardiovascular exercise, strength training, flexibility work, and mobility practices.

Timing your activity to enhance metabolic benefits while reducing injury risk is also key, as are recovery strategies that support your body's adaptation and prevent burnout. Effective plans incorporate gradual progression to improve fitness over time without hitting plateaus, and they prioritize enjoyment to help ensure long-term consistency.

A thoughtful, structured approach replaces the vague "exercise more" advice with practical, sustainable strategies tailored to your health goals and lifestyle.

Stress Resilience

Chronic stress affects nearly every system in the body, yet is often overlooked until stress-related conditions have already developed. A preventive approach to stress management begins with understanding your unique stress patterns and identifying the specific triggers that set them off.

This includes techniques to regulate your body's stress response, such as breathing exercises, meditation, and biofeedback. Cognitive strategies, like reframing unhelpful thought patterns, can reduce how intensely you react to stress.

Making changes to your environment to limit avoidable stressors, along with building a strong support network, also plays a key role in strengthening resilience.

This more complete approach treats stress not just as a psychological issue, but as a major contributor to physical illness. One that deserves early, proactive attention.

Sleep Optimization

Sleep quality plays a critical role in nearly every aspect of health, influencing immune function, cognitive performance, and metabolic balance. Despite its importance, most of us, including healthcare professionals, overlook sleep until serious disorders like apnea or insomnia are already present.

A preventive approach to sleep focuses on creating the right conditions for consistent, restorative rest. This includes practicing good sleep hygiene, aligning your sleep schedule with your natural circadian rhythms, and optimizing your environment, by adjusting light, temperature, sound, and air quality for ideal conditions.

Establishing calming pre-sleep routines helps the body transition smoothly from wakefulness to rest, while ongoing monitoring can reveal areas for improvement and help detect sleep-related conditions early.

By treating sleep as a foundation of preventive health rather than a secondary lifestyle concern, you support long-term well-being on multiple levels.

Oral-Systemic Integration

As explored in depth in Chapters 2 and 3, oral health has a direct and powerful influence on overall systemic health, making dental prevention a vital part of any comprehensive disease prevention strategy.

An effective oral-systemic approach begins with preventing periodontal disease, a major source of chronic inflammation that can affect the entire body. The frequency of professional dental cleanings should be tailored to your specific risk factors, rather than based on arbitrary timelines.

At home, using the right tools and techniques for your particular oral health needs is essential. It is equally important to establish the coordination between dental and medical professionals to ensure that oral conditions with potential systemic impacts are addressed collaboratively.

Monitoring inflammation through both oral and systemic markers, including the use of salivary diagnostics, adds another layer of insight. This integrated strategy helps close the longstanding divide between dental and medical care that persists in conventional healthcare, creating a more holistic and effective model of prevention.

Implementing Primary Prevention Strategies

Prevent disease before it starts, with smarter, personalized strategies.

True prevention begins long before symptoms appear. Focus on nutrition that matches your biology, movement that balances challenge and recovery, and stress strategies that build long-term resilience. Prioritize sleep as a foundation of health, not an afterthought, and treat oral health as a critical part of preventing systemic disease.

When personalized and coordinated, these core habits create the greatest impact on lifelong wellness. Long before medicine typically steps in.

Enhancing Secondary Prevention

Secondary prevention is the next step in prevention, including early detection and intervention of disease.

The Early Warning System

To optimize this crucial step in prevention, a more advanced approach is needed, one that goes beyond the basic screening tests used in conventional care. Standard screenings often identify problems only after they've progressed significantly.

In contrast, a more sophisticated "early warning system" involves expanded biomarker panels that pick up on subtle physiological changes, functional tests that assess how body systems perform under stress, and tools that detect early shifts before they cross diagnostic thresholds.

Similar to how we manage metrics within primary prevention, rather than relying on isolated lab values, this approach looks for patterns across multiple markers and tracks changes over time to catch concerning trends early. This transforms screening from a simple pass/fail model into a more nuanced and powerful tool for early intervention.

Jonathan recalled his experience that illustrates this distinction, "Standard blood work showed my thyroid levels 'within normal range' for years. But when I started working with a prevention-focused physician, we tracked patterns across multiple markers and identified early subclinical hypothyroidism despite my 'normal' TSH. Addressing this pattern early through targeted nutrition and supplements likely prevented full thyroid disease development."

The Personalized Screening Schedule

A more personalized approach recognizes that screening should be tailored to the individual rather than based on a one-size-fits-all model. This means adjusting the timing and frequency of screenings based on personal risk, with higher-risk individuals monitored more frequently.

It also involves using age-adjusted protocols that reflect biological age and overall health, rather than just chronological age.

Combining different screening methods can provide a fuller picture, while sequential testing, where follow-up tests are guided by initial results, adds precision to the process.

Finally, prioritizing screenings that offer the highest value for your specific situation helps ensure that time and resources are used wisely.

This individualized approach makes screening more effective, efficient, and relevant to your personal health profile.

Borderline Management

A proactive approach to screening focuses on addressing these warning signs before they become full-blown conditions. This includes developing intervention plans for borderline values instead of passively watching them worsen, prescribing targeted lifestyle changes that directly respond to early patterns, and increasing the frequency of monitoring for values that are moving in a concerning direction.

It also involves optimizing function in systems that are starting to show early signs of trouble and digging deeper to uncover the root causes behind unfavorable trends. By closing the gap between "normal" and "disease," this approach helps people take action when it can make the biggest difference, before small issues become serious health problems.

Diana highlighted this approach's value, recalling, "My liver enzyme values were 'within normal range' but trending worse over three years. Conventional doctors suggested waiting until they crossed diagnostic thresholds. My integrative provider instead implemented specific nutritional interventions targeting early inflammatory patterns. My values improved rather than continuing to deteriorate toward inevitable nonalcoholic fatty liver disease."

Optimizing Tertiary Prevention

Many chronic conditions tend to get worse over time if they aren't properly managed, but that progression isn't always inevitable. Preventing disease from advancing starts with regular checkups that use the right lab tests and health markers to track how things are going.

Taking action early, before a condition gets significantly worse, can make a big difference. The most effective strategies often combine treatment with lifestyle changes, like adjusting your diet, activity, or stress levels. Making changes to your environment to remove things that may speed up the condition, and staying connected with a strong support system, can also help you stick to your care plan.

This proactive approach challenges the common belief that chronic conditions will always get worse and shows that with the right steps, it is often possible to slow or even stop their progression.

Michael, diagnosed with early Parkinson's disease, experienced this distinction: "My initial neurologist focused exclusively on symptom management through medication, with the clear expectation of inevitable decline. My current doctor and movement disorder specialist instead implemented a comprehensive protocol including specific exercise, nutritional interventions, stress management, and carefully timed medication. Five years later, my function has remained stable rather than following the expected decline trajectory."

Building Powerful Prevention Partnerships With Your Providers

Putting comprehensive prevention into action requires more than personal effort. It depends on working effectively with your healthcare professionals.

While many clinicians are open to prevention, some may have limited training or experience with more advanced, proactive approaches. By taking a collaborative, respectful, and data-informed stance, you can turn even hesitant clinicians into valuable allies in your long-term health strategy.

Start by sharing your goals clearly and constructively. Bring in specific research or articles related to your prevention interests, and ask thoughtful, targeted questions that highlight areas for early action, such as lifestyle changes, functional testing, or expanded monitoring. Organize your priorities in writing, so your doctor understands your commitment and focus. When they show support or take steps in the right direction, express appreciation.

Framing your conversations around shared goals, like staying healthy, avoiding unnecessary treatments, or maintaining independence, builds trust and keeps the conversation productive, even if you have different starting points.

In addition to communication, make data your ally. Track how interventions, whether dietary changes, supplements, or medications, are affecting your key health markers. Share your results in a clear, organized way, so all your clinicians can see the impact and help refine your plan. Use agreed-upon measures to evaluate progress, and let the data, not just opinions, guide your decisions. Aligning on outcome ·goals and creating simple feedback loops helps your care team stay connected and focused on what works.

Another important benefit of using data in your prevention plan is that it can help ease any concerns your doctor may have about sharing health information they've generated. When you actively track and organize your own results, it reinforces your role as a responsible, engaged partner in your care. This often makes professionals more comfortable with open data sharing and supports your right to access and understand the full picture of your health.

By combining respectful education with clear, measurable results, you create a powerful partnership model that doesn't rely on authority or philosophy. Rather, it's built on shared purpose and real-world progress. This approach helps ensure that your prevention plan isn't just something you believe in, it's something your entire care team supports, monitors, and improves with you.

Action Items

As you get ready to learn how to effectively demand more from healthcare in the next chapter, consider taking these immediate actions to implement prevention oriented strategies:

1. **Establish your monitoring matrix** identifying which health markers you'll track, how frequently, and what represents optimal ranges rather than merely "normal" values.

2. **Implement one new primary prevention strategy** from one major category: nutrition, movement, stress management, sleep, or oral health. Start with one change, then add consecutive modest changes, that ultimately will build sustainable foundations.

Transformation develops gradually through consistent implementation rather than immediate overhaul. So, start where your motivation and resources allow while planning for more comprehensive implementation over time.

Prevention represents healthcare's greatest opportunity yet remains its most neglected dimension. By developing your own comprehensive prevention approach, you not only improve your personal health trajectory but also demonstrate to doctors what truly patient centered care should entail. Through this leadership, you contribute to the broader transformation of healthcare from disease management to health optimization, one professional relationship at a time.

Shift from waiting for illness to designing your wellness. Track your early health markers, audit your lifestyle habits, and start fixing risks before they become diseases.

Your health tomorrow is determined by your prevention choices today.

NINE

How to Demand More (and Get It)

"You can't always get what you want, but if you try sometimes, you might find, you get what you need." —Rolling Stones

Andrew had always been the ideal patient. He was punctual, polite, and passive. He accepted whatever care doctors offered without question, believing that challenging medical authority was inappropriate and possibly detrimental to his care. This approach seemed to work well enough, until his mother had her battle with cancer.

As he accompanied her to appointments, Andrew watched in dismay as she received convoluted care, minimal explanation of options, and treatments that sometimes seemed at odds with her goals and values. When complications developed, explanations were vague and dismissive. Questions were met with medical jargon rather than clear answers.

"One day, sitting in yet another waiting room, I had an epiphany," Andrew recalled. "My mother, who had been a forceful voice in every other area of life, had adopted the same passive patient role I had. We were behaving as if quality care was something to hope for rather than something to expect and require."

That realization transformed Andrew's approach. He began researching her condition extensively, taking detailed notes during appointments, requesting complete explanations of recommendations, and most importantly, clearly communicating expectations for care quality. When doctors didn't meet these expectations, he calmly but firmly requested adjustments. Ultimately he found different providers.

"The change was remarkable," Andrew explained. "Some doctors were initially defensive, but most responded positively once they understood we weren't challenging their expertise. The changes we made in doctors was essential to elevating my mom's treatment. The quality of care improved dramatically."

This experience permanently changed Andrew's approach to his own healthcare as well. "I realized that demanding more isn't about being difficult. It's about establishing appropriate expectations for something as important as healthcare. Doctors who truly prioritize patient wellness welcome engaged patients who hold them to high standards."

Andrew's story illustrates another core truth; the care you receive often reflects the care you expect and demand. While healthcare should consistently deliver excellence regardless of patient advocacy, the reality is that those who clearly communicate expectations and hold doctors accountable typically receive superior care.

In this chapter, you will find specific strategies for demanding more from healthcare. Not through confrontation or disrespect, but through clear communication, appropriate expectation setting, and effective advocacy when standards aren't met.

The Expectation Revolution

Healthcare operates on implicit assumptions that powerfully shape interactions between patients and doctors. Transforming these expectations represents the first and most fundamental step in demanding better care.

The Traditional Expectation Model

In conventional healthcare settings, many patient-provider relationships operate under a set of unspoken assumptions that tend to place patients at a disadvantage.

Patients are often expected to defer to doctor expertise without asking too many questions, while doctors typically control both the pace and content of appointments. Time constraints are frequently used to justify brief explanations, and treatment recommendations are often presented as decisions to accept rather than options to evaluate. Patients may feel discouraged from asking questions, especially if doing so seems to disrupt efficiency, and clinicians convenience often takes precedence over patient preferences. As a result, even superficial or perfunctory care is treated as acceptable.

These underlying dynamics create a power imbalance that limits communication, discourages collaboration, and ultimately prevents patients from receiving the thorough, personalized care they truly deserve.

The Partnership Expectation Model

Improving the quality of healthcare starts with redefining the expectations that shape the patient experience. At its core, healthcare should be a true partnership. One where both doctors and patients bring valuable expertise to the table.

Appointments should be structured around meeting patient needs, not just maintaining provider efficiency. Clear, thorough explanations and education aren't optional, they're essential for meaningful care.

Treatment decisions deserve careful, informed consideration, with patients fully understanding all available options before moving forward. Asking questions should be seen as a sign of thoughtful engagement, not a disruption to workflow. Patients' values and preferences should play a central role in shaping how care is delivered.

Above all, excellence in care should be the baseline, not a bonus. This new framework doesn't diminish the importance of clinician expertise; instead, it places that expertise within a collaborative model where patient authority is respected and actively supported.

The Care You Expect Shapes the Care You Get

Fair or not, healthcare often mirrors your level of engagement.

Patients who ask questions, set clear expectations, and speak up when something feels off don't just feel more in control, they usually get better care.

That's not how it should work.

But it's how it often does.

Until the system guarantees excellence for everyone, being an informed, assertive patient is one of your most powerful tools.

Communicating Expectations Effectively

As we have discussed, establishing a new, more collaborative set of expectations in your healthcare experience starts with clear, respectful communication that signals your desire to be an engaged partner in your care.

One effective approach is to strike a balance between appreciation and expectation. Begin conversations by genuinely acknowledging your professional's expertise, while also making it clear that you're seeking a partnership, not simply following instructions.

Preparing thoroughly for appointments demonstrates your commitment and sets the tone for meaningful collaboration. When asking questions, framing them as efforts to better understand, not to challenge, helps maintain trust and keeps the dialogue open.

Using collaborative language, such as "How can we approach this together?" instead of "What are you going to do?" reinforces the idea that you're both working toward the same goal. Keeping the focus on outcomes rather than specific methods also helps align perspectives and reduce tension.

This approach also acknowledges that you realize and accept that you are not just part of any care strategy, but you own your half of following through on any treatment recommendations that could affect the quality of your care.

Together, these techniques make it possible to assert your role in the care process without triggering defensiveness, laying the groundwork for a true partnership that supports better communication, decisions, and results.

Jennifer, who successfully transformed relationships with her healthcare team, described her approach: "I explicitly tell new doctors that I value their expertise and plan to be an engaged, informed participant in my care and that I will do my job to get the best results I can. I explain that I'll have questions, will want to understand options fully, and hope to make decisions collaboratively. This clarity from the beginning establishes the relationship I want, rather than defaulting to what I have experienced before."

The Information Demand Strategy

As we have discussed, complete, accessible information forms the foundation of quality healthcare but rarely arrives without specific, strategic requests. In this section we will cover specific, effective information demands that transform providers' communication patterns and dramatically improve care quality.

As with many sections of this book, use this section to capture what requests would be most helpful for your current situation and feel free to revisit it for more information when it is helpful in the future.

Full Disclosure Requests

Rather than accepting the limited information typically provided during appointments, use the following questions to explicitly request comprehensive disclosure for some commonly overlooked categories here:

- **Treatment option completeness**: "Are there any other approaches we haven't discussed yet, even if they're less common?"
- **Risk transparency**: "What are ALL the potential risks or side effects, even the rare ones?"
- **Evidence clarity**: "What's the quality of evidence supporting this recommendation? Are there any significant studies with different conclusions?"
- **Experience disclosure**: "What has your experience been with patients in similar situations who chose different options?"
- **Uncertainty acknowledgment**: "What aspects of my situation are you most uncertain about?"

These requests signal your expectation for complete information rather than simplified summaries, creating a more sophisticated and honest discussion.

Documentation Review Requests

While healthcare professionals typically control documentation content, you can significantly influence what appears in your records through strategic review:

- **Visit note requests**: "I'd like to review my appointment notes before they're finalized. Can you share a draft with me?"
- **Error correction initiation**: "I've noticed a few inaccuracies in my record that I'd like to correct. What's your process for making these adjustments?"
- **Addition requests**: "There are some important details missing from my history. Can we ensure these are documented properly?"
- **Rationale documentation**: "Would you mind documenting your reasoning for this recommendation in my record?"
- **Preference recording**: "Please note in my record that my preference is for conservative approaches whenever appropriate."

This documentation engagement ensures your record accurately reflects your history, concerns, and preferences rather than merely doctor impressions.

Brad, who discovered significant errors in his medical record, developed a proactive approach: "I now routinely request to review my visit notes within 48 hours of appointments. This simple practice has prevented numerous errors from becoming permanent parts of my record. Clinics initially seemed surprised by this request, but most now appreciate that it improves accuracy, or at least acknowledge that it helps them provide better care."

Test Result Ownership

Laboratory and imaging results offer vital insights into your health, far too important to be passively received or interpreted without your full understanding. To make these results truly useful, start by requesting complete access to your test data, not just simplified summaries like "normal" or "abnormal."

When reviewing results with your doctor, ask them to explain what they consider *optimal* ranges, as these are often more meaningful than the broad "normal" categories used by labs. If you're unfamiliar with the tests, request reference materials so you can better understand what each measurement reflects.

Ask how your current results compare with previous ones and whether any trends are starting to emerge. This turns isolated data points into a clear picture of your health over time. Finally, clarify what thresholds would trigger different treatment decisions so you can recognize when changes are meaningful.

Quality of Care Enforcement

Healthcare quality varies dramatically across doctors, facilities, and interactions. Establishing and enforcing clear quality guidelines significantly improves the care you receive.

Explicit Quality Expectation

Rather than simply hoping your healthcare professionals will meet your expectations, you can take a proactive role by clearly communicating what quality care looks like to you.

Letting your doctor know that you value a thorough, comprehensive assessment, rather than focusing solely on the most obvious explanations, sets the tone for deeper exploration. Expressing your preference for evidence-based care and asking to understand the strength of the evidence behind recommendations reinforces your desire for informed decision-making.

You can also emphasize the importance of care coordination by stating that you expect your doctors to communicate with one another and that you're willing to help facilitate that process.

If prevention is a personal priority, make it clear that you value early intervention and proactive strategies over reactive care. Finally, affirm your role in the care partnership by stating your expectation to be fully informed and actively involved in all decisions.

These types of statements help eliminate assumptions and establish a shared understanding, ensuring your clinician knows how to deliver care that aligns with your values and expectations.

Comparative Quality

Asking strategic, thoughtful questions is a powerful way to set a high bar for care while gathering meaningful insights for your decision-making. Rather than settling for whatever is offered, consider asking how the proposed approach compares to what's typically done at highly respected institutions.

This frames your care in a broader context of excellence. Inquire about outcomes directly, such as asking how your provider's success rates stack up against national averages.

Explore whether financial or institutional constraints might be shaping the recommendation by asking, "If resources weren't a factor, would you suggest a different approach?" You can also gain insight into best practices by referencing specialists, asking what experts who focus exclusively on this condition might recommend. Finally, invite your professional's personal perspective by asking what they would choose for themselves or a loved one in your situation.

This perspective not only helps surface valuable comparative information, but also signal that you're seeking optimal, not just adequate, care, reinforcing your commitment to thoughtful, informed choices.

> ## 📢 Don't Just Ask What, Ask Why Not?
>
> Sometimes the best care isn't offered first, it's filtered through cost, coverage, or institutional limits.
>
> Break through those barriers by asking:
>
> "If money or your system limits weren't a concern, would your recommendation change?"
>
> "What would a specialist, someone who sees this all day, every day, likely suggest?"
>
> "What would you choose for yourself or your family?"
>
> These aren't confrontational questions. They're clarifying tools, and they signal you're here for the best care, not just what's easiest to approve.

The Quality Feedback Loop

Recognizing excellence develops a cycle that helps create a culture where high-quality care becomes the norm. Providing specific, thoughtful feedback encourages doctors to continue what's working and consider where improvements could be made.

Positive reinforcement is powerful. For example, letting your doctor know that their detailed explanation of treatment options helped you make more informed decisions, reinforces the value of clear communication.

When offering suggestions, frame them constructively. You might mention that, in future appointments, you'd find it helpful to spend a bit more time reviewing test results in depth rather than just covering the basics.

Identifying patterns can also be helpful, such as noting that appointments often feel rushed toward the end and suggesting that slightly longer visits could allow for more comprehensive discussions.

Drawing from other experiences can offer perspective without criticism. For instance, explaining that a different doctor gave written summaries after visits and asking if something similar might also be possible.

Finally, normalizing your communication preferences can strengthen understanding, such as explaining that your questions come from a desire to learn and engage, not to challenge their expertise. This kind of specific, respectful feedback guides clinician behavior far more effectively than vague praise or general dissatisfaction, and it plays a meaningful role in improving care for everyone.

James, who systematically improved his healthcare experiences through feedback, shared his approach: "I make a point of specifically thanking doctors when they meet or exceed my standards. I also calmly note when my expectations aren't met, framing these observations as opportunities for improving our working relationship rather than complaints. Over time, this consistent feedback has transformed my care."

Insurance Medical Necessity Denials

Insurance companies frequently deny coverage for treatments providers recommend, citing "medical necessity" requirements. Here are some effective advocacy strategies that can often reverse these denials and secure appropriate coverage.

Documentation Enhancement Strategy

Many insurance coverage denials aren't due to actual ineligibility, but rather to incomplete or poorly documented information.

So, make sure your healthcare professionals clearly document the medical necessity of the treatment. This means requesting that their notes directly address the criteria insurers use to approve care. It's also important to include a full history of your condition in the supporting records, along with thorough documentation of any conservative treatments you've already tried and why they didn't work.

When possible, link the recommended treatment to specific functional limitations, such as difficulty walking or working, rather than just reporting discomfort or pain. If appropriate, having support from multiple providers can further reinforce the medical need.

With stronger documentation, you can turn borderline cases into clearly justified ones by giving insurance reviewers the specific, detailed evidence they need to approve coverage.

The Appeal Hierarchy Approach

Although insurance denials are often framed as final decisions, they rarely are. In many cases, persistence and strategy can make a significant difference.

One powerful option is to request a peer-to-peer review, where your doctor speaks directly with the insurance company's medical director to advocate for your case.

If the initial appeal is denied, don't stop there, as most plans offer multiple levels of appeal, and it's important to take full advantage of each one. When internal appeals are exhausted without success, you can escalate to an external review conducted by an independent party.

For denials that seem inappropriate or unjustified, involving your state's insurance regulatory agency may apply additional pressure. In more serious cases involving costly or critical care, seeking legal guidance can also be a valuable step.

By following this layered, step-by-step process, and combining it with strong documentation, you significantly increase your chances of overturning a denial and securing the care you need.

Elizabeth, who secured coverage for a specialized treatment after three denials, described her systematic approach: "I treated the appeal process like a project, understanding each level's requirements and decision criteria. I made sure our submissions precisely addressed the specific reasons cited for previous denials rather than simply resubmitting the same information. The third submission included additional research evidence, more detailed documentation of failed alternatives, and support from two additional specialists. This comprehensive approach finally got the care I needed approved."

The Medical Exception Request

When a recommended treatment falls outside standard insurance coverage guidelines, but is clearly the most appropriate option for your specific situation, submitting a medical exception request can often lead to approval.

The key is to highlight what makes your case different. Emphasize any unique medical characteristics or circumstances that set you apart from typical patients. Be sure to document any contraindications or risks associated with the treatments that are normally covered, making it clear why those options aren't suitable for you.

Supporting your request with relevant research that directly connects the proposed treatment to your condition adds credibility, and including a cost comparison may strengthen your case, especially if the requested treatment could ultimately reduce long-term expenses.

Finally, letters of support from multiple healthcare providers, written with clear and specific justification, can reinforce the medical necessity of your request. This approach respects the structure of insurance policies while presenting a strong case for why your situation merits an exception.

System Navigation Hacks

Healthcare systems develop bureaucratic processes that often impede optimal care. Strategic techniques can overcome these barriers and create more direct paths to quality care.

Gatekeeper Bypassing

Administrative gatekeepers often stand between patients and the decision makers who have the authority to resolve issues, but there are effective ways to navigate around these barriers.

One strategy is to respectfully request escalation by saying something like, "I understand you're not authorized to make exceptions to this policy. Could you connect me with someone who does have that authority?"

Another powerful approach involves documentation: ask the representative to note in your record that you requested a specific service, that it was denied for a specific reason, and that this information should be forwarded to the appropriate decision maker.

In some cases, it's more effective to step outside the typical communication channel altogether by contacting provider relations departments, patient advocacy offices, or even healthcare executives instead of relying on frontline staff. When time is a factor, clearly explain the urgency of the situation and why the standard timeline is not acceptable.

Using these strategies helps you move past roadblocks without confrontation, asserting your needs while keeping the focus on resolution.

Priority Signaling

Healthcare systems often manage appointments and service requests using rigid priority algorithms, rather than assessing each situation based on individual urgency. However, you can often improve response times by using strategic communication to signal your needs clearly and respectfully.

For example, requesting a specific timeframe helps set clear expectations: "Given the progressive nature of this condition, I need an appointment within the next two weeks. How can we make that happen?"

Articulating potential consequences also reinforces the importance of timely care: "If we delay addressing this issue, I'm concerned about [specific negative outcome]. How can we prevent that?" You can further strengthen your case by asking your doctor to include notes that document the time-sensitive nature of your condition.

Offering flexibility also helps: let staff know that you're available for last-minute cancellations and ask to be added to their call list.

Finally, acknowledging system pressures while expressing appreciation encourages cooperation: "I understand scheduling challenges, and I truly appreciate your help in finding a solution that prevents my condition from worsening." These respectful yet assertive approaches help ensure your care needs are recognized and prioritized within a constrained system.

Persistence

Healthcare bureaucracies often rely, sometimes unintentionally, on attrition, assuming that patients will eventually give up on legitimate requests out of frustration or exhaustion. The key to overcoming this barrier is structured persistence.

Start by setting up a consistent follow-up schedule to check on pending requests, and stick to it. Keep a detailed record of every interaction, including dates, names, and any promises made. Maintain a tone of pleasant persistence, respectful, but clearly showing that you're not going to let the issue drop.

Frame your communication as collaborative rather than confrontational, positioning yourself as someone who wants to work together to solve the problem rather than demanding special treatment. If progress stalls, don't hesitate to escalate appropriately within the organization, moving up the chain of command when necessary.

This structured, respectful persistence turns a single unanswered request into an ongoing process. One that often succeeds simply because you stay engaged when others might give up.

Charlie, who successfully navigated a complex insurance approval process, shared his approach: "I maintained a detailed log of every conversation, including who promised what and by when. In follow up calls, I specifically referenced these notes, which significantly increased accountability. I never expressed frustration even when it arose, instead consistently positioning myself as a partner in finding a solution. This systematic persistence eventually secured the specialized treatment I needed despite multiple initial denials."

Difficult Conversation Mastery

Healthcare inevitably involves challenging discussions about mistakes, disagreements, or substandard care. Handling these conversations effectively transforms potential confrontations into constructive problem solving.

Constructive Concern Expression

The way you communicate concerns in a healthcare setting can have a powerful impact on how your message is received and whether it's acted upon constructively. Framing your concerns thoughtfully helps maintain a collaborative relationship while still addressing issues clearly.

One effective approach is to raise questions that invite understanding rather than confrontation. For instance, expressing curiosity about why a particular decision was made when another option might align better with best practices.

Emphasizing shared goals also reinforces a sense of partnership, such as noting that you and your doctor both want a successful outcome and expressing concern that a specific issue could stand in the way. Sharing your personal experience honestly, describing how a situation made you feel and asking to prevent similar experiences in the future, creates empathy and mutual understanding.

Finally, acknowledging real-world constraints while suggesting ways to uphold care quality despite those challenges shows respect and willingness to collaborate.

These communication strategies help express valid concerns while avoiding defensiveness, ultimately strengthening the doctor-patient relationship.

Error Response Protocol

When mistakes happen in healthcare, your response can significantly influence not only how the issue is resolved but also the quality of your future care.

The most effective approach begins with calmly and clearly documenting what occurred, focusing on facts rather than assigning blame. When speaking with doctors or staff, frame your concern as a desire to understand: "I want to understand what led to [specific error] so we can prevent similar situations."

Keep the conversation centered on achieving the right outcome, not punishing someone for a mistake. If the issue appears to be the result of a broader process breakdown rather than an individual's actions, bring attention to the system as a whole.

You might ask, "What changes might help prevent this kind of situation for future patients?" This approach encourages constructive problem-solving, reduces defensiveness, and can improve not only your immediate care experience but also the system's ability to serve others more effectively.

⚒ Something Went Wrong?

Stay calm. Focus on what happened, not who's at fault.

Document the facts clearly.

When speaking with your doctor, try: "I'd like to understand what led to this so we can prevent it moving forward."

Focus on solutions, not blame.

Ask: "Is there a system change that might help future patients?"

A thoughtful response can improve your care and the system as a whole.

Partnership Optimization

As you have learned in Chapter 7, the quality of care you receive is deeply influenced by the strength of your relationship with your healthcare professional. Building a productive, lasting partnership starts with mutual respect, something that must be actively demonstrated on both sides.

While it's important to recognize the real-world constraints professionals face, like limited resources or scheduling pressures, those limitations shouldn't prevent you from expecting high-quality, thoughtful care.

When both patient and professional feel heard, respected, and equally engaged, the result is a relationship that supports better communication, greater trust, and consistently better health outcomes. So, now that you have assembled your optimized care team, use the following strategies to elevate the outcomes your team delivers.

Communication Preference Alignment

Miscommunication between patients and providers is a common, and often avoidable, source of frustration that can undermine even the most promising care relationships. Proactively aligning communication styles and expectations helps prevent these issues and improves outcomes.

Start by openly discussing how you best process information, for example: "I absorb things more clearly when I can see them written down. Could we use that approach when reviewing complex topics?"

Clarify how your professional prefers to handle questions and establish a clear protocol for follow-up communication. Finally, invite feedback to strengthen the relationship over time.

By being intentional and transparent, you create a stronger foundation for collaboration, reducing the chance of miscommunication and improving both the care experience and outcome.

Boundary Clarification

Unclear boundaries between patients and professionals can lead to confusion, frustration, and weakened partnerships. Setting clear, respectful boundaries helps both parties understand their roles and work together more effectively.

Again, affirm that while you deeply value your clinician's expertise and guidance, the final decisions about your care ultimately rest with you. Clarify when and how communication should happen, such as which issues warrant urgent contact and which can wait for scheduled appointments.

Express your expectation for full transparency by requesting complete information about your condition and available options, even if some details may be uncomfortable or unlikely.

Define how you want to participate in your care. For example, the fact that you would like to be actively involved in treatment planning while trusting your doctor's lead on technical procedures. Finally, establish a shared approach for handling disagreements by discussing how to navigate differing opinions constructively.

Setting these boundaries early on prevents the misunderstandings and unspoken assumptions that often erode trust and compromise care quality.

Katherine, who transformed a problematic doctor relationship into a productive partnership, described her approach: "Rather than switching doctors immediately when a significant problem arose, I initiated a direct conversation about how we can work together. I outlined specific communication preferences, clarified my desire for shared decision making, and proposed a more structured agenda to appointments. This open, honest discussion completely transformed our conversations from frustrating to highly productive."

Action Items

As you prepare to explore healthcare's technological future in the next chapter, consider taking these immediate actions to begin demanding more from your healthcare experiences:

1. **Create a personal expectation document** outlining your specific standards for provider communication, care thoroughness, partnership approach, and coordination. Leverage the content in this chapter to create a list of the most important topics, questions and statements to present to your personalized care team. Share this document with new doctors and review it with existing ones to establish clear expectations.

2. **Establish a feedback system** by documenting aspects of care that meet or exceed your standards, as well as areas for improvement, and communicating these observations to providers in a constructive, specific manner.

These actions continue to establish your role as an active participant in healthcare.

Healthcare excellence rarely arrives without setting clear guidelines and appropriate advocacy. By communicating your quality of care expectations, requesting complete information, addressing quality gaps, overcoming system barriers, and developing true partnerships, you transform from hoping for good care to ensuring it.

While the system rarely offers optimal care automatically, it typically responds to strategic direction. When you apply the communication frameworks outlined in this chapter, you transform standard care into precision-targeted treatment aligned with your goals.

Set clear expectations with every doctor you meet: partnership, full explanations, complete transparency. If they resist, move on. You are not begging for great care, you are leading it.

PART
IV

The Patient First Future

TEN

Interoperability, AI, and the Rise of Smart Care

"The future is already here—it's just not evenly distributed."
—William Gibson

When Melissa started experiencing crushing fatigue, brain fog, heart palpitations, and an overwhelming sense that something was deeply wrong, she was met with blank stares and vague reassurances.

"You're probably just stressed."

"Give it time."

"Your tests are normal."

But Melissa knew her body was not the same. Months after a mild COVID-19 infection, her life had changed, and not for the better.

Eventually, someone labeled it post-viral syndrome. A specialist called it long COVID. But no one could explain what was happening, or how to help.

"I was bouncing between a cardiologist, neurologist, pulmonologist, and psychiatrist," Melissa said. "Each one seemed to be working in a different world. No one saw me as a whole person. I felt lost in the system that was supposed to help me."

The emotional toll was staggering. Melissa didn't just feel sick. She felt invisible.

Desperate for answers, she made a decision: if the healthcare system couldn't connect the dots, she would.

She began digitizing everything; test results, symptom logs, imaging reports, appointment summaries, anything she could get her hands on. Using a personal health record app, she built a living health timeline that made sense of the chaos.

Then came the breakthrough. Melissa started visualizing her data: overlaying biomarker trends with her symptoms, mapping how medication changes aligned with good or bad days, and noting environmental triggers. Patterns began to emerge with clear, undeniable evidence that her experiences weren't random.

"When I showed these charts to my neurologist, she sat back in her chair and just stared for a moment," Melissa recalled. "She said, 'This changes how I see everything.' That moment gave me hope I hadn't felt in months."

But Melissa didn't stop there. She connected her doctors using secure communication tools, synced medication reminders with symptom tracking, and joined a digital community of patients navigating the similarly tangled mazes.

"Technology didn't replace my doctors, it gave them better insight," Melissa said. "I wasn't just managing my care anymore, I felt like I was shaping it. Where the system gave me fragments, I built a picture. Where I felt powerless, I found control."

Melissa's story reveals another uncomfortable truth; even the best doctors can't help when the system keeps them in the dark.

In this chapter, you'll discover how technology is reshaping what's possible in modern care and specific strategies for harnessing these innovations to improve your care, even before healthcare organizations fully embrace them.

The Interoperability Imperative

Healthcare's most persistent technological failure is the lack of seamless information exchange between different systems and clinicians, what experts call "interoperability." Despite decades of digitization, most healthcare data remains trapped in isolated systems that don't communicate effectively with each other.

These silos create significant problems for patients: duplicate testing, medication errors, missed connections between conditions, and the burden of repeatedly providing the same information to different providers. Yet, despite these obvious drawbacks, healthcare organizations have made only modest progress toward true interoperability.

The Interoperability Landscape

Understanding how healthcare information is currently shared reveals both serious challenges and promising opportunities. While Electronic Health Records (EHRs) have replaced paper charts with digital systems, they often make it difficult for different providers and institutions to share information smoothly.

Health Information Exchanges (HIEs) were developed to improve this by linking regional healthcare networks, but their effectiveness varies widely depending on the healthcare specialty, location and provider infrastructure. Patient portals give individuals limited access to their medical records, but these platforms often provide only partial information and lack advanced features.

On the technical side, FHIR standards (Fast Healthcare Interoperability Resources) are helping to create a shared language for health data, slowly improving connectivity between systems. In addition, as you learned in Chapter 4, recent Information Blocking Rules under the 21st Century Cures Act now require healthcare organizations to stop withholding health data that patients have a right to access.

Although these developments represent progress, they're unfolding gradually. In the meantime, patients need practical, immediate strategies to manage and unify their health information.

Personal interoperability, where you actively collect, organize, and share your own healthcare information, can help bridge the gaps in today's broken system and ensure your care is better connected.

Creating Personal Interoperability

Instead of waiting for healthcare systems to achieve seamless data sharing, you can take control by creating your own version of interoperability through strategic information management.

Start by collecting comprehensive records from all your providers, as outlined in Chapter 4, ensuring you have a complete view of your health history. Use personal health record platforms to organize and standardize this information, making it easier to access and share when needed.

Actively support communication among your care team by providing relevant documents or test results to each doctor, especially when systems don't automatically share data. For imaging, make sure to keep your own digital copies, so you're not dependent on slow or unreliable institutional transfers.

Use medication reconciliation tools to track prescriptions and dosages across different prescribers, reducing the risk of errors. Together, these steps create a patient-centered system that helps bridge the chasm left by institutional segmentation, improving coordination, safety, and outcomes in your care.

Daniel, who manages multiple chronic conditions, described his personal interoperability system: "I maintain all my medical and dental records in two different but connected apps on my phone, organized by condition, doctor, and date. I've created summary documents that extract key information in standardized formats. When seeing a new doctor, I share relevant summaries rather than expecting them to review hundreds of pages or waiting for official record transfers that often never arrive. This approach has prevented countless errors and additional, unnecessary work."

The Interoperability Advocacy Approach

You don't need to be a policy expert to help improve healthcare. Small, everyday actions can nudge the system in the right direction. For example, when switching doctors, ask for all of your records in digital form instead of paper. This encourages clinics to adopt modern, shareable formats that support better coordination.

When choosing a new healthcare professional or organization, ask whether they can easily share your records with other doctors. Providers that prioritize connected care are more likely to offer a smoother, safer experience. If poor record-sharing ever affects your treatment, don't hesitate to speak up. Giving feedback helps healthcare institutions understand the real-world consequences of disconnected systems.

If you're ever denied access to your own health records, you may be experiencing Information Blocking, something you have the right to report under the 21st Century Cures Act. You can also help by supporting patient advocacy groups working to improve how health data is shared and protected across the industry.

By taking these simple steps, you're not just improving your own care, you're helping create a more connected, patient-centered healthcare system for everyone.

The AI Revolution in Healthcare

Artificial intelligence and machine learning are transforming healthcare capabilities, creating opportunities for more precise, personalized, and predictive care. While institutional adoption remains uneven, patients can strategically leverage AI applications to enhance their healthcare experience.

The New Intelligence in Your Corner: How AI Is Quietly Empowering Patients

Artificial intelligence is no longer just a tool for researchers or large hospitals. It's quietly beginning to transform how patients understand their health, navigate decisions, and personalize their care in ways that were unimaginable just a few years ago.

Some of the most powerful advances are happening in areas like diagnosis and prediction. AI systems can now scan medical images or analyze lab results with remarkable precision, spotting patterns even expert clinicians might miss. These tools are already helping detect diseases earlier and more accurately, often before symptoms are obvious.

AI is also helping make sense of the overwhelming amount of information buried in medical records and scientific literature. With technologies like natural language processing, dense clinical notes can be distilled into meaningful insights, and relevant research can be surfaced quickly, even tailored to your specific condition.

Another breakthrough is happening in precision care. Instead of relying on one-size-fits-all treatments, AI can now help identify what's most likely to work for you based on your unique biology, lifestyle, and history. From adjusting medications to recommending therapies based on your genetics, these tools are beginning to make truly personalized medicine a reality.

And it's not just behind the scenes. Virtual assistants, powered by AI, can help you track symptoms, remind you to take medication, or guide you through decisions between visits. What once felt like isolated moments of care can now feel more continuous, connected, and responsive to your needs.

Bringing AI into Your Healthcare Journey

While many of the most advanced tools are still used in major hospitals and research centers, more and more AI-powered resources are becoming available to individuals and they're already making a difference.

Some people are turning to AI-based second opinion services, which review medical and dental records and test results with sophisticated algorithms to catch things that might have been missed. Others use smart symptom checkers that suggest possible causes based on your reported symptoms, helping you make more confident choices about when and where to seek care.

There are also tools that flag potential risks in your medication regimen, comparing prescriptions, over-the-counter drugs, and supplements to prevent dangerous interactions. And if you've ever tried to make sense of new research about your condition, AI can help with that too, connecting you with clinical trials or studies that match your unique health profile.

Zoe, a cancer patient, is one of many who have started to use these tools strategically. She recalled, "I also used a platform that analyzed my pathology data against thousands of similar cases to estimate how I might respond to different treatments. That information helped me ask better questions and work with my care team to make a plan I really understood."

What Zoe experienced is just the beginning. These tools aren't meant to replace your doctors, they're here to help you partner with them more effectively.

By using AI to gather insights, personalize decisions, and stay engaged between appointments, patients can become more informed, confident, and proactive.

Whether you're navigating a new diagnosis or managing a chronic condition, AI is beginning to offer something healthcare has long struggled to provide: clarity, connection, and control. Right at your fingertips.

The AI Discernment Framework

Not all healthcare AI tools are created equal. Some offer genuine value, while others may pose risks by providing inaccurate or poorly explained recommendations. To use AI effectively in your healthcare journey, it's important to evaluate these tools thoughtfully.

Start by checking whether the AI system has been properly validated against gold standard medical practices or peer-reviewed benchmarks. Tools that offer transparency clearly, explaining how they generate recommendations, are generally more trustworthy and easier to integrate into your decision-making.

Take time to understand what data the AI is using, whether it's drawing from your personal health records, population data, or other sources, as this affects the relevance and accuracy of its outputs. Be mindful of what the tool might *not* take into account, such as lifestyle factors, mental health status, or rare conditions that don't appear in standard datasets.

Finally, when bringing AI-generated insights to your doctor, present them as discussion points, not challenges to their expertise. Framing the information this way encourages collaboration and thoughtful consideration. By applying this kind of discernment, you can separate genuinely helpful AI tools from those that may offer little benefit, or even introduce confusion or risk.

The Remote Care Transformation

Telehealth and remote monitoring technologies have evolved from emergency pandemic measures to permanent healthcare delivery components. These approaches offer significant advantages for proactive, continuous care when strategically incorporated into your healthcare plan.

Strategic Telehealth Integration

Telehealth offers a wide range of opportunities to enhance your care, and understanding the different formats can help you take full advantage of what's available.

Synchronous video, popularized by products such as Zoom and FaceTime, facilitates real-time consultations with your clinician, making it easier to receive timely care without needing to travel. Asynchronous messaging, on the other hand, allows for nonurgent communication with your clinical team, letting you ask questions, request refills, or share updates without scheduling a full appointment.

Remote monitoring tools track your health data, such as blood pressure, glucose levels, or heart rate, between traditional visits, offering a clearer picture of how you're doing day-to-day.

Virtual second opinion services connect you with specialists from outside your geographic area, giving you access to broader expertise or providing care when your clinician is not available. Also, digital therapeutic programs can deliver structured, clinically backed interventions for managing conditions like anxiety, diabetes, or chronic pain.

By understanding the full spectrum of telehealth options, you can more effectively identify where remote care can support your specific health needs, improve convenience, and enhance outcomes.

James, who manages cardiac and respiratory conditions, described his telehealth strategy: "I've worked with my doctors to create a hybrid care model where in person visits focus on thorough physical examination and complex discussion, while regular video checkins address medication adjustments and manage my symptoms. I use remote monitoring to track key metrics daily, with algorithms flagging concerning patterns that trigger the clinical team to review. This approach has prevented at least one potential hospitalization by catching a problem before it became an emergency."

The Digital Therapeutic Revolution

Digital therapeutics, which are evidence-based, software driven interventions that prevent, manage, or treat medical conditions, represent some of healthcare's most significant emerging innovations. These digital interventions, when validated, offer new options for addressing many conditions, often with fewer side effects than traditional treatments.

The Digital Therapeutic Landscape

Digital therapeutics are reshaping how care is delivered, offering powerful tools that extend the benefits of treatment well beyond the doctor's office. From cognitive behavioral therapy apps that support mental health, to structured rehabilitation programs that help rebuild physical function, to chronic condition management platforms for diabetes or hypertension, these technologies provide structured, evidence-based support between clinical visits.

Some are even prescribed like medications, known as prescription digital therapeutics, and may be covered by insurance. Others focus on helping you build healthier habits, offering daily reinforcement to turn intentions into long-term change.

But not all digital health tools are created equal, and choosing the right ones requires a thoughtful approach. Before relying on any digital therapeutic, look for clinical evidence supporting its effectiveness. When possible, check if the product has received regulatory clearance, such as FDA approval, which signals a higher standard of review.

As always, ensure the platform is transparent about how it handles your personal health data, especially when sensitive information is involved. And most importantly, consider how it fits into your overall care plan. A good digital therapeutic should complement, not compete with, your doctor's guidance.

By seeking out tools that are not only convenient but also clinically effective, you can amplify your care between appointments and turn technology into a meaningful partner in achieving your goals.

Michelle, who struggled with insomnia for years, applied this framework successfully: "After trying various medications with troublesome side effects, I researched digital therapeutics for insomnia and identified a program with multiple randomized controlled trials demonstrating effectiveness. The structured six week protocol gradually retrained my sleep patterns through behavioral techniques delivered via my phone. My sleep improved significantly without the side effects I'd experienced with medications, and the program cost less than a single month of my previous prescription."

Provider Integration

Digital therapeutics offer the greatest impact when they're fully integrated into your overall care plan rather than used in isolation. To ensure this alignment, start by informing your healthcare providers about any digital tools you're using, so they're aware of how these interventions might influence your progress.

Share relevant data, such as outcomes, usage patterns, or symptom changes, so your care team can factor that information into clinical decisions. As digital therapies begin to show results, work with your professional to adjust medications or other treatments accordingly, avoiding unnecessary overlap or conflict.

It's also important to regularly assess whether the tool is helping you meet your goals, and to speak up if adjustments are needed. Ask your doctor to help tailor the digital therapeutic to your specific condition, preferences, or lifestyle.

Wearable Enhancement

Consumer health wearables have rapidly evolved from basic step counters into advanced health monitoring tools. When used strategically, they can shift from being simple fitness gadgets to powerful instruments that support your healthcare. Today's wearables can continuously track heart rate, detect irregular rhythms, analyze sleep patterns, monitor activity intensity and recovery, assess stress levels through heart rate variability, and even estimate metabolic responses to diet and exercise. By understanding what your device can do and discussing its features with your professional, you can choose a wearable that offers meaningful insights tailored to your health needs.

To move from curiosity to clinical relevance, it's important to use wearables systematically. Establish a baseline to understand your normal patterns, then track how your habits, environment, and interventions influence your readings.

Look for connections between your symptoms and specific data trends. Identify what tends to trigger flare-ups, and use the device to test how changes in behavior or treatment impact your results. This kind of structured use transforms passive monitoring into active health management.

For example, Brad, who lives with paroxysmal atrial fibrillation, collaborated with his cardiologist to use his smartwatch's ECG function regularly and during symptoms. He also tracked lifestyle factors like caffeine, alcohol, and sleep. Over six months, they identified that his episodes were most often triggered by poor sleep and dehydration. With this knowledge, he made targeted lifestyle adjustments and cut his episode frequency by 60%, without needing new medications.

To make wearable data truly useful for your healthcare professional, focus on clarity and relevance. Instead of sharing raw data, prepare a brief summary that highlights key patterns. Emphasize any links you've observed between symptoms and specific readings. Frame your insights as specific questions to guide discussion.

Visual formats, like graphs or charts, can make patterns easier to understand at a glance. And only share information that directly supports clinical decisions. With this approach, wearables can become not just devices you wear, but tools that empower your care.

Health Data Ownership

As healthcare technology generates increasingly comprehensive personal health information, data ownership and privacy considerations become crucial.

The Privacy-Utility Balance

Health data sits at the center of a delicate balance. It simultaneously has the power to improve care when used wisely, while also carries the risk of misuse if shared without clear boundaries. Navigating this tension starts with moving beyond all-or-nothing thinking.

Instead of sharing your full medical record with every entity that requests it, consider which specific data points are relevant to each situation and who truly needs access. Be clear about the purpose of why you are giving this data to your clinic.

Sharing should support defined, beneficial uses like treatment coordination, not vague or open-ended objectives.

Setting time limits, too, can be a valuable way to protect your data, so access to your information isn't indefinite. Keep in mind that healthcare providers also have rights, so if they need to maintain your data that has been shared with them, it may fall within their rights. Setting time limits can, however, be enforced in some instances and can certainly be applied to new health information that you accrue.

Understand when your data might be used in a de-identified form for research or analytics, and whether you're comfortable with that. In each decision, weigh the health benefits of sharing your data against your personal comfort level with privacy exposure.

Equally important is how consent is obtained. Traditional consent forms often rely on vague language and legalese, offering little clarity about what you're agreeing to. You have the right to ask for plain-language explanations that outline exactly what data will be shared, with whom, for what purpose, and for how long.

Rather than giving blanket permission, look for opportunities to authorize specific uses. Set expiration dates where possible and clarify whether the party you're sharing with will pass your data along to others (and to who).

When you approach data sharing with these principles in mind, you shift to protecting your privacy while still enabling the benefits of smarter, data-driven care.

Lauren, who participates in several digital health programs, described her approach: "I've created a personal data policy that I apply to all health technologies. I evaluate each service based on their patient controls, use limitations, and data security. I maintain a spreadsheet tracking exactly what information I've shared with which services, when that sharing authorization expires, and what specific uses I've permitted."

Navigating Smart Care Without Getting Exploited

As digital health tools become more prevalent, patients must take a few basic precautions to protect themselves. It's essential to read privacy policies thoroughly, especially those that involve data sharing or artificial intelligence, so you understand how your personal information may be used. Using strong passwords and enabling multi-factor authentication on any platform handling your health data is no longer optional but necessary. SMS texting and email are not secure, so avoid applications that rely solely on text and email for verification.

Your Data, Your Defense

Digital health tools offer power and convenience, but they also come with risks.

Protect yourself by doing what the system often doesn't:

- Read the fine print on data sharing and AI use

- Use strong passwords and turn on multi-factor authentication

- Avoid platforms that rely solely on text or email— they're not secure

In the digital age, privacy isn't automatic. It's something you have to actively protect.

Because once your health data is out, you can't pull it back.

Also, be wary of tools that lack clear business models or ask for excessive permissions without justification, and make it a habit to review your app settings regularly, revoking access to features you don't need.

Of course, the burden of safeguarding health data shouldn't fall entirely on patients. Yet in a system that still lacks consistent regulation and transparency, a measure of informed vigilance remains one of the few defenses available. Empowerment in this digital age includes knowing how to protect your autonomy, because smart care is only truly smart when it honors not just your data, but also your dignity and control as a patient.

Digital Health Ecosystem Navigation

The digital health landscape includes thousands of applications, devices, and platforms with varying quality, compatibility, and value. Seek to navigate this complex ecosystem in a way that maximizes benefits while minimizing wasted resources.

Digital Solution Selection

With so many digital health tools on the market, identifying which ones are truly worth your time and money requires a clear evaluation process. Start by making sure the tool directly addresses your specific health needs.

For example, a platform like *Cair* offers comprehensive support for dental care, while a tool like *SleepIQ* might be better suited for tracking sleep quality.

Usability also matters, no matter how advanced the features, a clunky or confusing interface will likely result in poor long-term engagement.

Finally, weigh the cost against the expected benefit. Some tools deliver high value for little to no cost, while others may charge premium prices without offering meaningful improvements.

With a little effort, you can cut through the hype and focus on digital health solutions that genuinely support your well-being.

Vicki, who once found managing multiple health apps overwhelming, discovered a game-changing solution through her primary care clinic. "My doctor's office started offering a digital platform that pulls together a lot of my information, including my glucose readings, blood pressure, fitness tracker, medications, and symptom logs. All in one place," she explained. "It's covered by the clinic, so it costs me nothing, but it gives me a full picture of my health that I never had before." The tool has helped Vicki spot trends and make better decisions. "Previously, I relied on a device that just tracked a few of my health metrics. Now, I won't use any app unless it provides a ton of value."

The Technology-Human Partnership

Digital health tools are most powerful when they complement, not replace, human clinical expertise. The key is striking the right balance.

Let technology handle what it does best: collecting data, spotting patterns, and organizing information for easier analysis. Then allow healthcare professionals to do what they're uniquely equipped for, making nuanced decisions, interpreting context, and building trust.

In the best care models, technology helps streamline and prioritize information so professionals can focus more deeply on patient care. It expands treatment options without undermining human judgment, and it supports, not disrupts, the therapeutic relationship between patient and doctor.

This balance isn't static; it should be revisited regularly to ensure that both tech and people are being used to their full potential.

Smart care is only truly smart when it respects your autonomy, not just your data.

Action Items

As we prepare to further explore the evolution from passive patient to empowered partner in the next chapter, consider taking these immediate actions to begin leveraging healthcare technology more effectively:

1. **Conduct a technology gap analysis** comparing your current digital health tools to the capabilities discussed in this chapter. Identify specific areas where additional technology might enhance your healthcare experience.

2. **Create your health data privacy framework** establishing personal guidelines for what information you'll share, with whom, under what circumstances, and with what limitations.

These steps begin transforming your relationship with healthcare technology to strategic utilization of digital capabilities that genuinely enhance your care. Through thoughtful implementation, rather than merely acquiring more technology, you can focus on meaningfully integrating these tools to support your goals.

Healthcare technology remains significantly fragmented and unevenly implemented across the system. However, individual patients who mindfully leverage available tools can create personal care experiences that anticipate where healthcare is gradually evolving. This includes connected, intelligent, personalized, and continuous care, rather than what the splintered, routine, homogenous, and episodic care we receive today.

The future of healthcare belongs to the informed and connected. Download your personal health apps today, including Cair. Consolidate your medical and dental records into a system you control. Don't wait for interoperability. Create it for yourself, right now.

ELEVEN

From Passive Patient to Empowered Partner

"The most common way people give up their power is by thinking they don't have any." —Alice Walker

When Carlos was diagnosed with Type 2 diabetes at 42, he did what most people instinctively do; he put himself completely in his doctor's hands.

"I just wanted someone to tell me what to do," he recalled. "I didn't know anything about diabetes. I figured if I just took the meds, showed up for appointments, and ate what they told me, I'd be fine."

At first, he diligently followed the advice. He took his metformin every morning, switched to a low-fat diet like the pamphlet recommended, and tried to walk for 30 minutes a few times a week. His doctor told him, "Just keep doing that, and we'll adjust your meds if needed." Carlos nodded obediently at every visit, trying to be the model patient.

But six months later, nothing had improved. His blood sugar readings spiked and crashed unpredictably. His weight barely budged. He was exhausted all the time, waking up soaked in sweat from blood sugar swings. At night, he lay in bed staring at the ceiling, wondering what he was doing wrong. His fingertips were sore from endless glucose checks. His ankles ached. The worst part was the creeping sense of helplessness.

"I was doing everything they told me to do, but it wasn't working," Carlos said. "And every time I went back, the answer was just more pills or higher doses. No one ever asked me what was happening in between visits."

Carlos hit his breaking point after one particularly grim appointment where a nurse practitioner told him, "Well, diabetes is progressive. You should expect it to get worse."

"No," Carlos thought fiercely as he walked to his car. "This can't be the whole story. I need to understand this for myself."

That night, he started researching. He read everything he could find, books like *Bright Spots & Landmines* by Adam Brown, forums on Diabetes Daily and articles from reputable sources like the American Diabetes Association and Mayo Clinic. He learned about the importance of carbohydrate counting, continuous glucose monitoring (CGM), and personalized nutrition, none of which had been emphasized by his original care team.

His "aha moment" came when he stumbled across a patient-led study showing how dramatically individualized responses to food could be, even so-called "healthy" foods like oatmeal could spike some people's blood sugar sky-high (Zeevi et al. 2015).

"They're treating me like a textbook case," Carlos realized, "but I'm not a textbook."

Armed with new knowledge, Carlos found a new physician, a young endocrinologist who, in their first meeting, listened carefully instead of lecturing.

"Here's the deal," Carlos said, sliding a battered notebook across the table. "I've been tracking everything; meals, exercise, sleep, stress, you name it. I'm not looking for someone to tell me what to do. I'm looking for a partner."

The doctor smiled and said, "Good. That's exactly how it should be."

Together, they developed a plan: Carlos started low-carb, high-protein meal planning, began using a CGM to spot hidden blood sugar spikes, and fine-tuned his medication based on daily trends rather than monthly lab reports.

Carlos's tracking system became a lifeline. He logged:

- Every meal and snack (with carb counts)
- Blood sugar readings (before and after meals)
- Exercise sessions (type, duration, and intensity)
- Sleep hours and quality
- Stress levels (rated on a 1–10 scale)

He organized it all into simple spreadsheets, color-coded by category, with weekly charts he brought to his doctor's appointments. He could now see, not guess, what triggered spikes, like noticing that even "healthy" whole-grain wraps sent his numbers soaring, while a spinach omelet kept him stable.

Within three months, his A1c dropped by nearly two points, he needed half the medication, and he felt like he finally had his life back. But the biggest shift wasn't on paper, it was in his mindset.

"I wasn't just a guy with a disease anymore," Carlos said. "I became the manager of my own health, with the experts I chose helping me, not controlling me."

Carlos's story captures exactly what this book is about: transforming from a passive patient into an empowered partner. As you prepare to put each phase you have learned about into action, remember that every step, from getting your records, building your team, tracking your data, standing up for yourself, to using technology wisely, will help you, as it helped Carlos, reclaim control.

Carlos didn't reinvent medicine. He simply refused to settle for being a spectator in his own declining care. And that one decision changed everything.

What started with confusion and frustration turned into clarity, momentum, and genuine partnership. His outcome didn't come from luck or privilege. It came from learning to ask better questions, track what mattered, and expect more from the people guiding his care.

That power is not unique to Carlos.

If you've read this far, it's because you're ready to step into that same role.

Maybe something in your care didn't sit right. Maybe a diagnosis felt rushed, a bill didn't make sense, or you had the sinking sense that you weren't being heard; just processed.

You started asking questions. And the more questions you asked, the more you uncovered.

That's what this book has been about; pulling back the curtain. You've seen misaligned incentives, the bureaucratic roadblocks, the siloed systems, and the language designed to confuse you.

But now you've seen what else is possible.

This chapter isn't about new information. It's about a new identity.

Because information only becomes power when you act from it. And action only becomes lasting when it's aligned with how you see yourself.

So here's the shift: You are no longer a passive patient. You are a partner. A planner. A leader.

You command your healthcare experience. Not because the system suddenly got easier, but because you no longer give away your authority within it.

Understanding This Shift

For years, most of us were taught, subtly or overtly, to defer in healthcare. We sit quietly in the waiting room. We nod while the doctor speaks, even though we are overwhelmed. We walk out with instructions we don't understand, and then blame ourselves if outcomes fall short.

But that's not care. That's compliance.

Empowerment doesn't mean confrontation. It doesn't mean challenging every diagnosis or rejecting every plan. It means holding your healthcare professionals to a higher standard of collaboration and holding yourself to a new standard of participation.

You don't have to know everything to ask better questions. You don't have to fix the system to take charge of your experience within it. You just have to decide: *I won't go unheard in this space again.*

Power Without Permission

One of the most liberating things you'll discover is that no one needs to grant you the right to lead your care. You can stop waiting for permission and start organizing your health around your values, your questions, and your clarity.

That starts with your records. They are no longer abstract data points held in someone else's system. They are your history, your evidence, your foundation. When you've seen how your information is scattered, ignored, or distorted, you realize how crucial it is to claim and curate it. Not just for reference, but for strategy.

When your information becomes your tool, not your barrier, everything shifts. You stop repeating yourself across offices. You stop accepting vague summaries. You begin spotting contradictions, trends, and omissions that others miss. And when you bring that insight into the exam room, the power dynamics shift, without you ever raising your voice.

Your care becomes *co-designed*. Not dictated. Not assumed.

Assembling Alignment

You've also learned something vital: your health is not just the sum of specialists and appointments. It's a system you live in. One that you can choose to design more intentionally.

Building a true care team isn't about collecting credentials. It's about choosing partners who respect your role in your own well-being. Some of the most important decisions you'll ever make won't be about treatments. They'll be about people: who you trust, who listens, who collaborates, and who doesn't.

This chapter isn't about naming names or chasing the "best doctor." It's about recognizing that the most skilled clinicians may still be a poor fit if they dismiss your concerns, fail to coordinate with others, or leave you feeling more confused than confident.

Great care doesn't happen in isolation. It's built through relationships. Relationships you intentionally shape. That might mean asking your doctor to communicate with your dentist. It might mean switching specialists. It might mean insisting on clarity when vague answers are offered.

It always means remembering: **you are the only one present at every healthcare decision made about you. You are the constant.** Everyone else is temporary.

The Quiet Radicalism of Prevention

We tend to think of prevention as something passive; floss more, eat better, move a bit. But you've now seen how prevention is actually a radical act of self-leadership. It defies the industry's focus on interventions and complexity. It says, "I will not wait for damage to react. I will invest in the conditions that help me thrive."

And it's not just about avoiding illness. It's about building vitality, resilience, and clarity. The kind of health that makes you more capable in every part of your life.

What does prevention look like now?

It looks like tracking patterns before symptoms emerge. It looks like investing in your oral health as a gateway to systemic wellness. It looks like understanding your unique risks and moving from general advice to personalized strategy. It looks like keeping your information organized, your questions prepared, and your focus long-term.

And most of all, it looks like knowing that quality healthcare doesn't begin at the doctor's office. It begins with you.

A New Kind of Confidence

The more you see how the system works (and doesn't) the more you might feel overwhelmed. That's normal. But confidence isn't the absence of complexity. It's the decision to proceed anyway. On your terms.

You don't need to know everything. You just need to start asking:

- What do I want from this interaction?
- What's missing from this picture?
- Who else needs to be looped in?
- How will I follow up?

This kind of thinking isn't reserved for experts. It belongs to anyone who's decided that passivity is no longer enough.

Your Role Has Changed

If this book has done its job, it hasn't just informed you. It has **rewritten the role you see yourself playing**.

You're no longer an observer of your own care. You're the point of integration. The connector. The translator. The memory. The advocate.

When systems break down, you step in. When communication fails, you initiate. When decisions get rushed, you slow them down.

You've seen too much to play small now.

You Are the Standard

What you expect from your care will shape the care you receive. Providers and systems will rise to the standard you hold. Or they will be replaced. That isn't arrogance. That's leadership.

If your presence in an exam room, phone call, or billing dispute helps one healthcare professional remember the kind of partnership they once went into medicine to offer, you've changed more than your outcome. You've shifted the system. Even if just a little.

And if enough of us do this, if we stop complying with dysfunction, and start insisting on collaboration, the system can't help but evolve.

This Is Not the End

This chapter is not a conclusion. It's a checkpoint.

Ahead of you is a path defined not by guarantees, but by greater agency. You will still face challenges. You will still encounter confusion, resistance, and indifference. But you won't be approaching those moments the same way you did before.

You'll ask different questions. You'll set clearer boundaries. You'll expect more. And accept less. You'll advocate with purpose, not apology.

Because you've crossed the line that matters most: You've stopped waiting for care. You've started commanding it.

And from here, that changes everything.

You're Not Waiting for the Future. You Create It.

When Sarah first opened this book, she felt like she was drowning. With three chronic conditions and a history of complicated surgeries, her medical records were scattered across twelve clinics in three different states. Her appointments left her feeling rushed and confused, often walking out with more questions than answers. Despite spending over $4,000 annually on premiums for her "comprehensive" insurance plan, she faced unexpected bills totaling $7,300 in the last year alone. Paperwork consumed her kitchen table, and anxiety about her next medical encounter kept her awake at night.

"I felt powerless," she recalled, tears welling up as she described those dark days. "Like I was caught in a system designed to process me and there was nothing I could do about it. My health was deteriorating, and I couldn't even get straight answers about my treatment options."

Today, Sarah's healthcare experience looks dramatically different. Her transformation began with a single, determined step. Over three weeks, she methodically collected every test result, diagnosis, and treatment record, organizing them into a comprehensive digital file she controls. This information foundation changed everything.

Now, Sarah arrives at appointments with a clear agenda and prepared questions. She records key conversations (with permission) and takes detailed notes. She researches treatment options thoroughly before making decisions. Her prevention plan is more robust than anything her doctors had suggested. And she's saved $5,800 in unnecessary procedures and billing errors this year by understanding and questioning charges.

"The system hasn't changed," Sarah notes with a confident smile, "but my experience has transformed completely. I'm no longer at the mercy of a broken system. Last month, when a specialist tried to dismiss my concerns, I simply pulled up my symptom tracker showing a clear pattern he'd missed. His face immediately changed. For the first time, I felt like an equal partner in my care. That moment alone was worth every hour I spent organizing my records."

Sarah's transformation captures the central message of this book: When you control your records, understand your options, and leverage your data effectively, you don't need to wait for healthcare reform to experience better care.

Overcoming Common Obstacles

Perhaps you're thinking:

"I don't have enough time for this." Consider this, the average person spends about 17 hours annually dealing with healthcare paperwork and billing issues. Implementing these strategies requires about 20 hours upfront, then saves you around 15 hours every subsequent year, not counting the time saved avoiding unnecessary appointments and treatments.

"I'm intimidated by healthcare professionals." You don't need confrontation skills to be effective. The quiet, prepared patient using the documentation methods outlined within this book and at **unfaircare.com/resources** often achieves better results than someone more assertive but less organized.

"My situation is too complex." Complex health situations actually benefit most from these approaches. The more doctors involved, the more critical it becomes to have someone (you) maintaining the complete picture.

"I'm not sure I can do this." Start small. Request just one set of records. Complete just one provider assessment. Each small success will build your confidence for the next step.

Envision Your Transformed Healthcare Experience

Imagine walking into your next appointment completely prepared. You have questions ready, understand your options, and know exactly what information you need. Rather than feeling rushed and confused, you feel centered and in control.

Picture having your complete records accessible during an emergency, potentially saving crucial minutes and preventing dangerous treatment errors.

Visualize the satisfaction of partnering with doctors who respect your engagement, the kinds of relationships that emerge when you demonstrate your commitment to collaborating in your care.

This isn't fantasy. It's the reality experienced by those who have implemented these strategies.

Your Impact Extends Beyond Your Care

When you transform your healthcare experience:

1. **You influence providers** who experience the value of collaborative relationships with informed patients
2. **You help family members** who learn from your example how to become active participants in their own care
3. **You impact institutions** that gradually adapt their practices in response to patient expectations
4. **You contribute to cultural change** that redefines what healthcare can and should be

True healthcare empowerment is not just a personal benefit, it's a form of leadership that creates ripples throughout the system.

Your Personal Commitment

Before closing this book, complete this simple commitment:

Today, I will take this one specific action to begin my healthcare transformation:

I'm doing this because:

The person who will support me in this journey is:

I will check my progress on (date):

One Year Later

One year after implementing these strategies, Sarah faced a new diagnosis. But this time, everything was different. She had her complete history at her fingertips. She knew which questions to ask and how to research her options thoroughly. Her primary doctor and specialist communicated effectively because she facilitated their connection. She understood her insurance coverage before making treatment decisions. And when a billing error occurred, she resolved it with a single email rather than months of frustration.

"The diagnosis was still scary," Sarah reflected, "but I never felt helpless or alone. I had the tools and confidence to navigate every step of the process. That made all the difference."

The healthcare landscape will continue to evolve through policy changes, technological innovations, and organizational restructuring. But you don't have to wait for these large-scale transformations to improve your own care.

Your health is too precious to entrust to a system designed to serve interests other than your own. You have the right and the ability to demand better, to create better, and to experience better. Your health data belongs to you. Claim it, understand it, and use it.

Healthcare is not something that happens to you. It is something you help create, one decision, one demand, one action at a time.

The age of passive patients is over. The era of empowered partners has begun.

And it begins with you. Today.

References

American Cancer Society (ACS). 2022. *Limitations of Mammograms*. Atlanta, GA: American Cancer Society. https://www.cancer.org /cancer/types/breast-cancer/screening-tests-and-early-detection /mammograms/limitations-of-mammograms.html.

American Cancer Society (ACS). 2023. *Cancer Facts & Figures 2023*. Atlanta, GA: American Cancer Society. https://www.cancer.org /content/dam/cancer-org/research/cancer-facts-and-statistics/annual -cancer-facts-and-figures/2023/2023-cancer-facts-and-figures.pdf.

Anderson, Gerard F. 2007. "From 'Soak the Rich' to 'Soak the Poor': Recent Trends in Hospital Pricing." *Health Affairs* 26 (3): 780–789. https://doi.org/10.1377/hlthaff.26.3.780.

Armfield, Jason M. 2010. "Development and Psychometric Evaluation of the Index of Dental Anxiety and Fear (IDAF-4C+)." *Psychological Assessment* 22 (2): 279–287. https://doi.org/10.1037/a0018678.

Beaton, Laura, Ruth Freemen, Gerry Humphris. 2014. "Why Are People Afraid of the Dentist? Observations and Explanations." *Medical Principles and Practice* 23 (4): 295-301. https://doi.org/10.1159/000357223.

Centers for Disease Control and Prevention (CDC). 2024. *Fast Facts: Health and Economic Costs of Chronic Conditions*. Atlanta, GA: U.S. Department of Health and Human Services. https://www.cdc.gov /chronic-disease/data-research/facts-stats/.

Centers for Medicare & Medicaid Services (CMS). 2023. *National Health Expenditure Data: Historical.* U.S. Department of Health and Human Services. https://www.cms.gov/research-statistics-data-and -systems/statistics-trends-and-reports/nationalhealthexpenddata /nationalhealthaccountshistorical.

Chen, Lena M., Wildon R. Farwell, and Ashish K. Jha. 2009. "Primary Care Visit Duration and Quality: Does Good Care Take Longer?" *Archives of Internal medicine* 169(20): 1866–1872. https://doi .org/10.1001/archinternmed.2009.341

Ciatto, Stefano, Nehmat Houssami, Daniela Ambrogetti, Rita Bonardi, G. Collini, and M. R. Del Turco. 2007. "Minority report— false negative breast assessment in women recalled for suspicious screening mammography: imaging and pathological features, and associated delay in diagnosis." *Breast Cancer Res Treat* 105 (1): 37–43. https://doi.org/10.1007/s10549-006-9425-3.

CRICO Strategies. 2015. *Malpractice Risks in Communication Failures: 2015 Annual Benchmarking Report.* Boston, MA: CRICO Strategies. https://www.rmf.harvard.edu/Malpractice-Data/Annual-Benchmark -Reports/Risks-in-Communication-Failures.

Cutler, David M. 2021. *The Quality Cure: How Focusing on Health Care Quality Can Save Your Life and Lower Spending Too.* Oakland, CA: University of California Press.

DesRoches, Catherine M., Jan Walker, Leonor Fernandez, Suzanne Leveille, Tom Delbanco, and Sigall K. Bell. 2019. "OpenNotes After 7 Years: Patient Experiences With Ongoing Access to Their Clinicians' Outpatient Visit Notes." *Journal of Medical Internet Research* 21 (5): e13876. https://doi.org/10.2196/13876.

Deyo, Richard A., Sohail K. Mirza, Judith A. Turner and Brook I. Martin. 2009. "Overtreating Chronic Back Pain: Time to Back Off?" *Journal of the American Board of Family Medicine* 22 (1): 62–68. https://doi.org/10.3122/jabfm.2009.01.080102.

Dominy, Stephen S., Casey Lynch, Jiyoun Ermini, Malcolm Benedyk, Adeel Marczyk, Trucchi Konradi, Marcia Nguyen, et al. 2019. "*Porphyromonas gingivalis* in Alzheimer's Disease Brains: Evidence for Disease Causation and Treatment with Small-Molecule Inhibitors." *Science Advances* 5 (1): eaau3333. https://doi.org/10.1126/sciadv .aau3333.

Gooch, Kelly. 2016. "Medical Billing Errors Growing, Says Medical Billing Advocates of America." *Becker's Hospital Review.* https://www .beckershospitalreview.com/finance/medical-billing-errors-growing -says-medical-billing-advocates-of-america/.

Hajishengallis, George. 2015. "Periodontitis: From Microbial Immune Subversion to Systemic Inflammation." *Nature Reviews Immunology* 15 (1): 30–44. https://doi.org/10.1038/nri3785.

Hashimoto, Motomu, Toru Yamazaki, Masahide Hamaguchi, Takeshi Morimoto, et al. 2015. "Periodontitis and Porphyromonas gingivalis in Preclinical Stage of Arthritis Patients." PloS one, 10(4), e0122121. https://doi.org/10.1371/journal.pone.0122121.

Health Care Cost Institute. 2023. *Facility Fees and How They Affect Health Care Prices.* Washington, DC: Health Care Cost Institute. https: //healthcostinstitute.org/images/pdfs/HCCI_FacilityFeeExplainer.pdf.

Himmelstein, David U., Terry Campbell, and Steffie Woolhandler. 2020. "Health Care Administrative Costs in the United States and Canada, 2017." *Annals of Internal Medicine* 172 (2): 134–142. https://doi.org/10.7326/M19-2818.

Institute of Medicine (IOM). 2013. *Best Care at Lower Cost: The Path to Continuously Learning Health Care in America*. Washington, DC: The National Academies Press. https://doi.org/10.17226/13444.

Institute of Medicine (IOM). 2003. *Unequal Treatment: Confronting Racial and Ethnic Disparities in Health Care*. Edited by Brian D. Smedley, Adrienne Y. Stith, and Alan R. Nelson. Washington, DC: The National Academies Press. https://doi.org/10.17226/10260.

Jeffcoat, Marjorie K., Robert L. Jeffcoat, Patricia A. Gladowski, James B. Bramson, and Jerome J. Blum. 2014. "Impact of Periodontal Therapy on General Health: Evidence from Insurance Data for Five Systemic Conditions." *American Journal of Preventive Medicine* 47 (2): 166–174. https://doi.org/10.1016/j.amepre.2014.04.001.

Liu, Cheng, Chengcheng Gong, Shuai Liu, Yingjian Zhang, Yongping Zhang, Xiaoping Xu, et al. 2019. "18F-FES PET/CT Influences the Staging and Management of Patients with Newly Diagnosed Estrogen Receptor-Positive Breast Cancer: A Retrospective Comparative Study with 18F-FDG PET/CT." *The Oncologist* 24 (12): e1277–e1285. https://doi.org/10.1634/theoncologist.2019-0096.

Makary, Martin A., Michael Daniel M. 2016. "Medical error—the third leading cause of death in the US." *BMJ (Clinical research ed.)* 353 (i2139). https://doi.org/10.1136/bmj.i2139.

Mehrotra, Ateev, Eric T. Roberts, J Michael McWilliams. 2017. "High-Price And Low-Price Physician Practices Do Not Differ Significantly On Care Quality Or Efficiency." *Health affairs (Project Hope)* 36(5), 855–864. https://doi.org/10.1377/hlthaff.2016.1266.

Michalowicz, Bradley S., James A. Hodges, Thomas P. DiAngelis, Raymond P. Lupo, John P. Novak, Heather Ferguson, Steven A. Buchanan, et al. 2006. "Treatment of Periodontal Disease and the Risk of Preterm Birth." *New England Journal of Medicine* 355 (18): 1885–1894. https://doi.org/10.1056/NEJMoa062249.

Mitchell, Jean M. 2008. "Utilization Trends for Advanced Imaging Procedures: Evidence From Individuals With Private Insurance Coverage in California." *Medical Care* 46(5):p 460-466. https://doi .org/10.1097/MLR.0b013e31815dc5ae.

Nasseh, Kamyar, Barbara Greenberg, Marko Vujicic, and Michael Glick. 2014. "The Effect of Chairside Chronic Disease Screenings by Oral Health Professionals on Health Care Costs." *American Journal of Public Health* 104 (4): 744-750. https://doi.org/10.2105/AJPH.2013 .301644.

Nasseh, Kamyar, Marko Vujicic, and Michael Glick. 2017. "The Relationship between Periodontal Interventions and Healthcare Costs and Utilization. Evidence from an Integrated Dental, Medical, and Pharmacy Commercial Claims Database" *Health Economics* 26 (4): 519–527. https://doi.org/10.1002/hec.3316.

National Cancer Institute. 2023. *SEER Cancer Stat Facts: Female Breast Cancer*. Bethesda, MD: Surveillance, Epidemiology, and End Results (SEER) Program. https://seer.cancer.gov/statfacts/html/breast.html.

National Institutes of Health (NIH). 2023. *TMJ Disorders*. National Institute of Dental and Craniofacial Research. https://www.nidcr.nih .gov/health-info/tmj.

Offenbacher, Steven, Vern Katz, Gregory Fertik, John Collins, Doryck Boyd, Gayle Maynor, Rosemary McKaig, James Beck. 1996. "Periodontal Infection as a Possible Risk Factor for Preterm Low Birth Weight." *Journal of Periodontology* 67 (10s): 1103–1113. https://doi.org/10.1902/jop.1996.67.10s.1103.

Office of the U.S. Surgeon General. 2022. *Addressing Health Worker Burnout: The U.S. Surgeon General's Advisory on Building a Thriving Health Workforce.* Washington, DC: U.S. Department of Health and Human Services. https://www.hhs.gov/surgeongeneral/priorities /health-worker-burnout/index.html.

Patient Rights Advocate (PRA). 2023. *The Fourth Semi-Annual Hospital Price Transparency Compliance Report.* Newton, MA: Patientrightsadvocate Org Inc. https://www.patientrightsadvocate. org/february-semi-annual-compliance-report-2023.

Ponemon Institute. 2016. *Electronic Health Records (EHR) and Healthcare IT: The Hidden Costs and Productivity Losses.* Traverse City, MI: Ponemon Institute. https://www.ponemon.org/library/electronic -health-records-ehr-and-healthcare-it-the-hidden-costs-and -productivity-losses.

Schwartz, Lisa M., and Steven Woloshin. 2019. "Medical Marketing in the United States, 1997–2016." *JAMA* 321 (1): 80–96. https://doi.org /10.1001/jama.2018.19320.

Shrank, William H., Teresa L. Rogstad, and Natasha Parekh. 2019. "Waste in the US Health Care System: Estimated Costs and Potential for Savings." *JAMA* 322 (15): 1501–1509. https://doi.org/10.1001 /jama.2019.13978.

Simpson, T. Campbell, Jo C Weldon, Helen V Worthington, Ian Needleman, Sarah H Wild, et al. 2015. "Treatment of Periodontal Disease for Glycaemic Control in People with Diabetes Mellitus." *The Cochrane database of systematic reviews*, 2015(11), CD004714. https://doi.org/10.1002/14651858.CD004714.pub3.

Sinsky, Christine, Lacey Colligan, Ling Li, Mirela Prgomet, Sam Reynolds, Lindsey Goeders, Johanna Westbrook, Michael Tutty, and George Blike. 2016. "Allocation of Physician Time in Ambulatory Practice: A Time and Motion Study in 4 Specialties." *Annals of internal medicine* 165(11): 753–760. https://doi.org/10.7326/M16-0961.

Sjögren, Petteri, Erika Nilsson, Marianne Forsell, Olle Johansson, and Janet Hoogstraate. 2008. "A Systematic Review of the Preventive Effect of Oral Hygiene on Pneumonia and Respiratory Tract Infection in Elderly People in Hospitals and Nursing Homes: Effect Estimates and Methodological Quality of Randomized Controlled Trials." *Journal of the American Geriatrics Society* 56 (11): 2124–2130. https://doi.org/10.1111/j.1532-5415.2008.01926.x.

Schneider, Eric C., Arnav Shah, Michelle M. Doty, Roosa Tikkanen, Katharine Fields, Reginald D. Williams II. 2021. "Mirror, Mirror 2021 — Reflecting Poorly: Health Care in the U.S. Compared to Other High-Income Countries." *Commonwealth Fund*, Aug. 2021. https://doi.org/10.26099/01dv-h208.

Tilburt, Jon C., Matthew K. Wynia, Robert D. Sheeler, Bjorg Thorsteinsdottir, Katherine M. James, Paul S. Egginton, and Megan Allyse. 2013. "Views of US Physicians About Controlling Health Care Costs." *New England Journal of Medicine* 369 (7): 566–574. https://doi.org/10.1056/NEJMsa1205098.

Tonetti, Maurizio S., and Thomas E. Van Dyke. 2013. "Periodontitis and Atherosclerotic Cardiovascular Disease: Consensus Report of the Joint EFP/AAP Workshop on Periodontitis and Systemic Diseases." *Journal of Clinical Periodontology* 84 (4S): S24–S29. https://doi.org /10.1902/jop.2013.1340019.

Walker, Jan, Tom Delbanco, Joann G. Elmore, Richard M. Ralston, Sigall K. Bell, Suzanne Leveille, Joann D. Stametz, et al. 2010. "Open Notes: Doctors and Patients Signing On." *Annals of Internal Medicine* 153 (2): 121–125. https://doi.org/10.7326/0003-4819-153-2 -201007200-00008.

Wall, Thomas, and Marko Vujicic. 2015. "Emergency Department Use for Dental Conditions Continues to Increase." *Health Policy Institute Research Brief*. American Dental Association. https://mediad. publicbroadcasting.net/p/wusf/files/201802/ADA.pdf.

Zafar, S. Yousuf, Jeffrey M. Peppercorn, Deborah Schrag, Donald H. Taylor, Amy M. Goetzinger, Xiaoyin Zhong, Amy P. Abernethy. 2013. "The Financial Toxicity of Cancer Treatment: A Pilot Study Assessing Out-of-Pocket Expenses and the Insured Cancer Patient's Experience." *The Oncologist* 18 (4): 381–390. https://doi.org/10.1634 /theoncologist.2012-0279.

Zeevi, David, Tal Korem, Niv Zmora, David Israeli, Daphna Rothschild, Adina Weinberger, Orly Ben-Yacov, et al. 2015. "Personalized Nutrition by Prediction of Glycemic Responses." *Cell* 163 (5): 1079–1094. https://doi.org/10.1016/j.cell.2015.11.001.

Zimmerman, Sheryl, Philip D. Sloane, Kimberly Ward, et al. 2020. "Effectiveness of a Mouth Care Program Provided by Nursing Home Staff vs Standard Care on Reducing Pneumonia Incidence A Cluster Randomized Trial." *JAMA Network Open* 3(6)e204321.

Appendices & Extras

Your First 10 Moves After Reading Unfair Care

Don't just close this book. Close the gap between broken care and empowered care, starting today. Here's exactly where to begin:

1. Request Your Full Medical Records

From your primary care doctor and any specialists you've seen in the last 3 years.

2. Request Your Full Dental Records Through the Cair App

Consolidating and protecting your records in one place you control. Just go to cair.net or scan the QR code below:

235

3. Audit Your Health Bills

Review your past 3 healthcare bills. Request itemized statements. Challenge any errors.

4. Create Your Emergency Dossier

A simple one-page document containing essential information for crisis care.

5. Choose Your Core Care Team

Identify your primary care physician, dentist, and key specialists you trust. Then confirm they communicate to each other.

6. Schedule a Prevention-First Visit

Book an appointment that focuses purely on wellness, not sickness, including dental, medical, or both.

7. Prepare Your Empowered Patient Script

- Practice asking doctors:
- "Can you explain that decision?"
- "What are my other options?"
- "How can I access my full records today?"

8. Know Your Rights

Learn your rights under HIPAA and the 21st Century Cures Act (In Appendix G, with additional resources available at **unfaircare.com /resources**).

9. Demand Cost Transparency

Before accepting any procedure or test, ask for clear, written cost estimates and authorization requirements.

10. Tell One Person About *Unfair Care*

Share what you've learned. Start a ripple effect. Empowerment spreads. And it starts with you.

The Essential Healthcare Documents

Effective healthcare management requires several key documents that facilitate information sharing, ensure appropriate care during emergencies, and protect your preferences when you cannot actively communicate. Creating and maintaining these documents represents a fundamental component of healthcare empowerment.

1. Your Health Summary Document

This one to two page document provides essential information for new providers or emergency situations:

Key Components:

- Demographic information and emergency contacts
- Current medical and dental conditions with diagnosis dates
- Past major surgeries or hospitalizations with dates
- Current medications with dosages and prescribing doctors
- Medication and contrast allergies with specific reaction descriptions
- Implanted devices or artificial joints
- Primary care physician and key specialist contact information

Strategic Use:

- Provide to new providers before initial appointments
- Carry a copy during travel in case of emergency care needs
- Update quarterly or whenever significant changes occur
- Share with family members or healthcare proxies

Sample Format:

HEALTH SUMMARY FOR: Jane M. Smith

DOB: 05/15/1972 | EMERGENCY CONTACT: John Smith (Husband) 555-123-4567

CURRENT CONDITIONS:
- Hypothyroidism (diagnosed 2015)
- Mild Hypertension (diagnosed 2019)
- Periodontal Disease (diagnosed 2018)
- Migraine with aura (diagnosed 2007)

SURGICAL HISTORY:
- Laparoscopic cholecystectomy (2016)
- C-section delivery (2003)

CURRENT MEDICATIONS:
- Levothyroxine 88mcg daily (Dr. Wilson)
- Lisinopril 10mg daily (Dr. Wilson)
- Sumatriptan 50mg as needed for migraine (Dr. Chen)
- Vitamin D3 2000IU daily (OTC)

ALLERGIES:
- Penicillin (hives and facial swelling)
- Iodine contrast (nausea, vomiting)

PROVIDERS:
- Primary Care: Dr. Sarah Wilson, Internal Medicine (555-234-5678)
- Neurology: Dr. Michael Chen (555-345-6789)
- Dentistry: Dr. Robert Johnson (555-456-7890)

ADDITIONAL NOTES:
- Titanium dental implant position #19 (2020)
- Family history of cardiovascular disease (father, brother)

2. Advance Directive

This legal document, to be prepared by an attorney, specifies your healthcare preferences should you become unable to communicate decisions personally:

Key Components:

- Living will section detailing treatment preferences in various scenarios
- Healthcare proxy designation naming individuals authorized to make decisions on your behalf
- Specific guidance regarding life sustaining treatments
- Values statement explaining your general healthcare philosophy
- Witnessing or notarization according to state requirements

Strategic Considerations:

- Review state specific requirements as laws vary significantly
- Discuss your preferences thoroughly with designated proxies
- Distribute copies to proxies, primary care provider, and specialists

- Store in easily accessible location known to family members
- Review and update after major life events or every 3-5 years

3. HIPAA Authorization

This document specifies who may access your protected health information:

Key Components:

- Designated individuals authorized to receive your health information
- Specific information types they may access
- Time limitations (if any) on authorization
- Revocation provisions
- Your signature and date

Strategic Uses:

- Authorize family members to discuss your care with doctors
- Enable non-spouse partners to participate in healthcare discussions
- Allow adult children to assist with healthcare management
- Facilitate care coordination across doctors

4. Medication Management Document

This comprehensive medication record provides more detail than the brief summary:

Key Components:

- Complete list of prescription medications, over-the-counter drugs, and supplements
- Dosages, frequencies, and administration instructions
- Start dates and, if applicable, end dates
- Prescribing doctors
- Purposes for each medication
- Previously tried medications with reasons for discontinuation
- Noted side effects or concerns

Strategic Uses:

- Bring to all appointments regardless of specialty
- Review during medication reconciliation
- Reference when considering new medications
- Update immediately upon any prescription changes

5. Symptom and Reaction Log

This document tracks symptoms, treatment responses, and patterns over time:

Key Components:

- Symptom descriptions with specific details
- Timing information (onset, duration, frequency)
- Severity ratings using consistent scales (e.g. 1-10)
- Associated factors (activities, foods, stressors, etc.)
- Treatment responses
- Pattern observations
- Create visuals whenever possible (graphs, etc.)

Strategic Uses:

- Identify triggers and exacerbating factors
- Evaluate treatment effectiveness
- Recognize patterns not obvious in isolated observations
- Provide objective data for appointment discussions
- Support medical necessity documentation for treatments or accommodations

Essential Questions for Healthcare Providers

The questions you ask significantly influence the information you receive and the care you ultimately experience. The following question frameworks will help elicit comprehensive information across various healthcare scenarios.

1. New Provider Interview Questions

When selecting new healthcare professionals, these questions help assess compatibility with your partnership expectations:

Partnership Approach:

- "How would you describe your approach to working with patients who want to be actively involved in their care decisions?"
- "What's your perspective on patients who research their conditions and bring information to appointments?"
- "How do you handle situations where patients might disagree with your recommendations?"

Communication Style:

- "What's your typical approach to explaining complex medical information?"
- "How do you prefer to be contacted between appointments for nonurgent questions?"
- "What's your policy on sharing test results? Do patients receive them directly or only after your review?"

Care Coordination:

- "How do you typically communicate with other professionals involved in a patient's care?"
- "What role do you see yourself playing in coordinating care across specialties?"
- "How do you handle situations where specialists might recommend conflicting approaches?"

Practice Logistics:

- "What's your typical response time for patient messages or portal communications?"
- "How does your practice handle appointment scheduling for urgent concerns?"
- "What's your approach to prescription refills and medication adjustments between visits?"

2. Diagnosis Discussions

When receiving new diagnoses, these questions help ensure comprehensive understanding:

Condition Basics:

- "Could you explain exactly what this condition is and how it typically affects people?"
- "What likely caused or contributed to this condition in my specific case?"
- "How might this condition evolve over time? What's the typical progression?"

Diagnostic Certainty:

- "How confident are you in this diagnosis? What other conditions might present similarly?"
- "What additional testing, if any, might help confirm or clarify this diagnosis?"
- "What signs or symptoms would suggest we should reconsider this diagnosis?"

Treatment Considerations:

- "What are ALL the treatment options available, from most to least aggressive?"
- "For each option, what are the potential benefits and risks or side effects?"
- "How quickly do we need to make treatment decisions?"

Practical Implications:

- "How might this condition and its treatment affect my daily activities?"
- "What lifestyle modifications might help manage this condition?"
- "What specific signs or symptoms should prompt me to seek immediate medical attention?"

3. Treatment Decisions

When considering treatment options, these questions help evaluate alternatives comprehensively:

Evidence Assessment:

- "What evidence supports this treatment approach for someone with my specific characteristics?"
- "How long has this treatment been available, and how has its long term effectiveness been evaluated?"
- "Are there any ongoing studies or recent developments that might affect treatment recommendations?"

Outcome Expectations:

- "What specific improvements might I realistically expect from this treatment?"
- "How long typically before results become noticeable?"
- "What percentage of patients experience significant improvement with this approach?"

Alternative Evaluation:

- "What other approaches might address this condition, even if they're less commonly used?"
- "How does this recommendation compare to alternatives in terms of risks, benefits, and evidence quality?"
- "What happens if we delay treatment or choose nonintervention at this time?"

Personalization Factors:

- "How does my specific situation influence the appropriateness of this treatment?"
- "Would your recommendation be different if I were older/younger/had different comorbidities?"
- "If this were your own health situation or that of a close family member, would your thinking change in any way?"

4. Medication Discussions

When considering new medications, these questions help understand implications comprehensively:

Medication Basics:

- "What exactly does this medication do in the body, and how does that help my condition?"
- "Is this medication treating the underlying condition or managing symptoms?"
- "Is this the newest option, the most established option, or somewhere in between?"

Administration Details:

- "What's the optimal timing and method for taking this medication?"
- "How might food, other medications, or activities affect how this medication works?"
- "What should I do if I miss a dose?"

Effect Expectations:

- "How quickly should I notice the effects from this medication?"
- "What positive effects indicate the medication is working properly?"
- "What side effects might occur, and which would warrant contacting you?"

Long Term Considerations:

- "Is this medication typically used short term or long term?"
- "Are there concerns about tolerance, dependence, or diminishing effectiveness over time?"
- "What monitoring will we do to evaluate this medication's effectiveness and safety?"

5. Tests and Procedures

When considering diagnostic tests or procedures, these questions help understand purpose and implications:

Necessity Assessment:

- "How will this test or procedure change my treatment or management plan?"
- "What specific information will this provide that we don't already have?"
- "Are there alternative ways to obtain this information with less risk or cost?"

Process Understanding:

- "Could you walk me through exactly what happens during this test/procedure?"
- "What preparation is required beforehand, and what recovery should I expect afterward?"
- "Who specifically will be performing this test/procedure and interpreting the results?"

Risk Evaluation:

- "What are the common and rare risks associated with this test/procedure?"
- "How frequently do complications occur, and what's done to minimize those risks?"
- "Are there specific risks in my case given my history and condition?"

Results Interpretation:

- "When and how will I receive the results?"
- "What range of potential findings might we see, and what would each suggest?"
- "If results are inconclusive, what would be the next steps?"

Negotiation Scripts for Healthcare Challenges

Effective negotiation often requires language that balances assertiveness with collaboration. The following scripts provide starting points for addressing common healthcare challenges.

1. Insurance Denial Appeals

When coverage is denied for recommended care:

Initial Phone Appeal: "I'm calling regarding claim #[number] which was denied on [date]. I've reviewed the denial reason, and I believe additional information might change this determination. My doctor has documented this treatment as medically necessary because [specific clinical justification]. Could you please explain exactly what additional documentation would help demonstrate that this meets your coverage criteria?"

Written Appeal Follow Up: "I'm writing to appeal the denial of coverage for [treatment/service] (claim #[number]). This treatment was recommended by Dr. [name] based on [specific medical findings] and is supported by [clinical guidelines/research evidence/prior treatment failures]. Enclosed please find additional documentation including:

1. A letter from Dr. [name] explaining the medical necessity
2. My relevant medical records demonstrating [qualifying condition/symptoms]
3. Research literature supporting this approach for my specific situation
4. Documentation of previous treatments that proved ineffective

I request reconsideration of this denial based on the enclosed information demonstrating that this treatment meets your stated coverage criteria for medical necessity. Please provide your determination in writing within [timeframe specified in policy]."

2. Medical Record Correction Requests

When errors appear in your medical records:

Verbal Request: "I've reviewed my medical record from my visit on [date], and I noticed some information that needs correction for accuracy. On page [number], it states [incorrect information], but the accurate information is [correction]. Could you please explain your process for correcting this information to ensure my record is accurate?"

Written Follow Up: "I am writing to request a correction to my medical record from my appointment on [date]. The current record contains the following inaccuracy:

Current statement: [quote exact language] Requested correction: [specific correction]

This correction is important because [reason that affects treatment decisions or creates misleading impressions about your health]. Under HIPAA, I have the right to request amendment of inaccurate information in my health records. Please process this correction within 60 days as required by federal regulations and provide written confirmation when completed."

3. Appointment Access Negotiations

When facing long wait times for needed appointments:

Urgent Situation: "I understand you're scheduling [specialist] appointments for [distant date], but my situation has some urgency due to [specific reason, including worsening symptoms, impact on function, treatment planning needs]. Dr. [referring physician] considers this time sensitive because [specific clinical reason]. Could you please check for any cancellations or work me into the schedule sooner? I can be available on short notice if that helps."

Waitlist Request: "Since the next available appointment is [distant date], I'd like to be placed on your cancellation list for earlier openings. My schedule is flexible on [days/times], and I can arrive within [timeframe] of notification. Could you please make a note of this in your scheduling system and let me know how your cancellation process works?"

Physician-to-Physician Request: "Given the scheduling delay, would it be possible for my primary physician, Dr. [name], to speak directly with [specialist] about my case? Perhaps a brief physician-to-physician consultation could determine whether my situation warrants earlier evaluation or if there are interim steps we should take while waiting for the appointment."

4. Cost Transparency Discussions

When seeking clarity on healthcare costs:

Preservice Inquiry: "I'm scheduled for [procedure/service] on [date], and I need to understand the complete costs involved before proceeding. Could you provide a written estimate that includes all charges, including the facility fee, professional services, anesthesia if applicable, and any equipment or supply charges? Also, could you verify whether all providers involved are in network with my insurance [plan details]?"

Billing Department Negotiation: "I've received a bill for [amount] for [service]. This amount is more than I can pay at once due to [brief explanation if appropriate]. I'd like to discuss either a discount for prompt payment or an interest-free payment plan. Many facilities offer discounts of 20-30% for direct patient payment. What options do you have available for patients in my situation?"

Surprise Bill Challenge: "I've received a bill for [service] performed by [provider] during my [procedure] on [date]. Before my procedure, I confirmed that the facility and primary provider were in network with my insurance. I was not informed that out of network providers would be involved or given an opportunity to request in network alternatives. Under the No Surprises Act, I believe this may qualify as a protected surprise bill. Could you please review this and explain how we can resolve it within network benefit levels?"

5. Treatment Alternative Discussions

When proposing alternatives to recommended treatments:

Research Based Alternative Request: "Thank you for recommending [treatment]. I've done some research and found that [alternative approach] might also be effective for my condition, potentially with [fewer side effects/lower cost/better alignment with my preferences]. Studies by [researcher/institution] suggest [brief evidence summary]. Would you be willing to discuss this alternative and whether it might be appropriate in my specific case?"

Stepped Approach Negotiation: "I understand you're recommending [aggressive treatment] for my condition. Given my [specific concerns, including side effect risks, cost, recovery impact], I'm wondering if we might consider a stepped approach, starting with [less aggressive option] and monitoring closely for [specific timeframe]. If we don't see [specific improvement markers], I'd be willing to proceed to more aggressive treatment. Would this approach be medically reasonable in my situation?"

Complementary Approach Integration: "In addition to the conventional treatment you've recommended, I'm interested in incorporating [complementary approach] which has shown some evidence for [specific benefit] in patients with my condition. Would you be comfortable with me pursuing this alongside conventional treatment, and could you advise on any potential interactions or monitoring we should consider?"

Healthcare Tracking Tools

Effective health management requires systematic tracking of various factors affecting your wellbeing. The following frameworks provide starting points for developing personalized tracking systems.

1. Symptom Tracking Matrix

This comprehensive approach captures detailed patterns about symptoms:

Key Tracking Categories:

- **Date and Time:** When exactly symptoms occur
- **Symptom Description:** Specific characteristics and location
- **Severity Rating:** Consistent scale (typically 1-10)
- **Duration:** How long symptoms persist
- **Preceding Factors:** Activities, foods, stressors, etc. before onset
- **Alleviating Factors:** What helps reduce symptoms
- **Exacerbating Factors:** What makes symptoms worse
- **Associated Symptoms:** Other issues that occur simultaneously
- **Intervention Responses:** Effects of medications or other treatments

2. Medication Effect Monitoring

This tracking system helps evaluate medication impacts comprehensively:

Key Tracking Elements:

- **Medication Details:** Name, dose, timing, adjustments
- **Target Symptom Measurements:** Changes in the issues being treated
- **Side Effect Monitoring:** Emergence and patterns of unwanted effects
- **Interaction Observations:** Effects when combined with other treatments
- **Adherence Documentation:** Consistency in taking as prescribed
- **Circumstantial Variations:** Different effects under different conditions

Implementation Options:

- Dedicated medication tracking apps with reminder functions
- Spreadsheet with daily documentation and trend graphing
- Printed calendar with color coded notation system
- Combined with symptom tracking in integrated health journal

3. Lifestyle Correlation System

This approach identifies relationships between behaviors and health outcomes:

Key Tracking Categories:

- **Nutrition Patterns:** Food types, timing, quantities
- **Sleep Metrics:** Duration, quality, consistency
- **Physical Activity:** Type, intensity, duration, frequency
- **Stress Levels:** Perceived intensity and sources
- **Environmental Exposures:** Weather, allergens, pollutants
- **Health Markers:** Symptoms, energy, mood, measured biomarkers

Analysis Approach:

- Identify patterns connecting specific behaviors with health changes
- Establish baseline relationships during stable periods
- Test hypotheses through deliberate modifications
- Document time relationships (immediate vs. delayed effects)
- Note interaction effects between multiple factors

4. Treatment Outcome Evaluation

This framework systematically assesses intervention effectiveness:

Key Evaluation Dimensions:

- **Target Symptom Changes:** Primary issues the treatment addresses
- **Functional Improvements:** Daily activity and quality of life impacts
- **Side Effect Development:** Unwanted consequences
- **Adherence Challenges:** Difficulties following treatment as prescribed
- **Satisfaction Assessment:** Subjective experience with the treatment

- **Cost-Benefit Evaluation:** Value relative to money and time investments

Implementation Timeline:

- Establish clear pretreatment baseline measurements
- Document immediate effects during initial implementation
- Evaluate short term impacts at 2-4 weeks
- Assess medium term outcomes at 2-3 months
- Conduct long term evaluation at 6-12 months

5. Provider Interaction Documentation

This system creates accountability and continuity in healthcare relationships:

Key Documentation Elements:

- **Appointment Details:** Date, provider, primary purpose
- **Questions Prepared:** Issues you planned to address
- **Information Provided:** What the provider communicated
- **Recommendations Made:** Specific advice or instructions
- **Decisions Reached:** Mutual agreements about next steps
- **Outstanding Questions:** Issues requiring further clarification
- **Follow Up Plans:** Scheduled actions and responsibilities

Strategic Applications:

- Review before subsequent appointments for continuity
- Reference when inconsistencies arise between providers
- Use to track recommendation implementation
- Evaluate patterns in provider care quality and communication over time
- Support appeals or complaints when necessary

Healthcare Financial Management Tools

Navigating healthcare finances requires specific approaches for understanding, planning, and optimizing healthcare spending.

1. Healthcare Budget Framework

This structured approach helps plan for healthcare expenses:

Fixed Healthcare Costs:

- Insurance premiums
- Membership fees for direct primary care or concierge services
- Ongoing prescription medications
- Regular preventive care appointments
- Chronic condition management visits
- Necessary medical supplies

Variable Healthcare Expenses:

- Deductible funding based on historical utilization
- Typical copayment and coinsurance amounts
- Anticipated specialist visits
- Projected diagnostic testing
- Seasonal medication needs
- Expected dental procedures

Emergency Healthcare Reserves:

- Deductible and out-of-pocket maximum coverage
- Non-covered service allowance
- Out-of-network care possibilities
- Travel healthcare considerations
- Coverage gap protection

Tax Advantaged Funding Strategies:

- Health Savings Account (HSA) contributions
- Flexible Spending Account (FSA) allocation
- Health Reimbursement Arrangement (HRA) utilization
- Premium tax credit optimization
- Medical expense tax deduction planning

2. Bill Review Protocol

This systematic approach helps identify and address billing errors:

Verification Steps:

1. Confirm service dates match actual appointments
2. Verify all listed services were actually provided
3. Check for duplicate charges for single services
4. Confirm provider names and credentials are accurate
5. Verify coding matches diagnoses and services received
6. Compare charges against your benefit structure
7. Check for appropriate insurance adjustments

Common Error Types:

- Unbundling (charging separately for elements of a single procedure)

- Upcoding (using higher level service codes than provided)
- Balance billing for in network services
- Missing contracted discounts
- Incorrect patient information affecting coverage
- Missing prior authorization notations
- Incorrectly applied deductibles or out-of-pocket limits

Resolution Approach:

1. Document specific errors identified
2. Contact billing department with precise details
3. Request itemized explanation of all charges
4. Ask for supervisor review for complex issues
5. Submit formal appeal with supporting documentation
6. Request written confirmation of corrections
7. Verify adjustments on subsequent statements

3. Insurance Optimization Framework

This approach helps select and utilize health insurance effectively:

Plan Selection Factors:

- Premium costs relative to expected utilization
- Provider network inclusion of your preferred healthcare team
- Specific coverage for your known health conditions
- Prescription formulary alignment with your medications
- Deductible and out-of-pocket maximum levels
- Special program availability for your health situations

Utilization Optimization:

- Preventive service identification (typically covered at 100%)
- In network provider verification before receiving care

- Prior authorization requirement adherence
- Referral process compliance when required
- Prescription tier optimization strategies
- Appeal process utilization for inappropriate denials

Coverage Gap Strategies:

- Supplement identification for routine excluded services
- Direct pay negotiation approaches for non-covered care
- Manufacturer assistance programs for medications
- Charitable foundation resources for specific conditions
- Medical tourism options for major procedures
- Community and government program eligibility assessment

4. Medical Debt Management System

This framework helps address healthcare financial challenges:

Prevention Strategies:

- Cost estimation before receiving nonemergency care
- In network confirmation for all care team members
- Charity care or financial assistance application before services
- Payment plan negotiation prior to treatment
- Deposit and payment expectation clarification
- Alternative treatment option exploration when appropriate

Negotiation Approaches:

- Prompt pay discount requests (typically 10-30%)
- Itemized bill review for error identification
- Comparable cost research for leverage
- Hardship adjustment requests with documentation

- Interest-free payment plan proposals
- Lump sum settlement offers at reduced amounts

Resolution Pathways:

- Hospital financial counseling services
- Patient advocate assistance programs
- Medical billing advocate engagement
- Nonprofit credit counseling services
- Legal aid for medical debt issues
- Bankruptcy protection evaluation for catastrophic situations

APPENDIX G

Healthcare Rights Reference Guide

Understanding your legal rights enables more effective navigation of the healthcare system. This guide summarizes key healthcare rights under U.S. law.

1. Information Access Rights

HIPAA Right of Access:

- Right to inspect and obtain copies of your health records
- Records must be provided within 30 days (with possible 30 day extension)
- Fees limited to reasonable, cost-based amounts
- Right to request records in specific formats when feasible
- Right to have records sent directly to designated third parties

21st Century Cures Act Provisions:

- Prohibition on Information Blocking by healthcare providers and IT vendors
- Right to access electronic health information without delay
- Right to access health information through smartphone apps using standardized interfaces

- Protection against excessive fees for electronic health information access

Informed Consent Requirements:

- Right to receive information about proposed treatments in understandable terms
- Disclosure of risks, benefits, and alternatives before consenting
- Opportunity to ask questions before making decisions
- Right to refuse recommended treatments
- Ongoing consent process rather than one time documentation

2. Privacy and Confidentiality Rights

HIPAA Privacy Protections:

- Right to know how your health information is used and disclosed
- Right to request restrictions on certain uses and disclosures
- Right to confidential communications through alternate means or locations
- Right to be notified of privacy breaches involving your information
- Right to file complaints about privacy violations

Special Category Protections:

- Enhanced privacy for mental health treatment records
- Additional protections for substance use disorder treatment information under 42 CFR Part 2
- Genetic information protection under GINA
- State specific protections that may exceed federal requirements
- Minor privacy rights that vary by state and treatment type

Disclosure Limitations:

- Requirement for minimum necessary information disclosure
- Restricted access to psychotherapy notes
- Authorization requirements for marketing purposes
- Limitations on disclosure for research without specific consent
- Restrictions on disclosure to employers without authorization

3. Quality and Safety Rights

Treatment Standards:

- Right to care meeting professional quality standards
- Protection against abandonment once care relationship established
- Right to appropriate pain assessment and management
- Right to care free from discrimination based on protected characteristics
- Right to second opinions and provider changes

Hospital Specific Rights:

- Right to know identity and role of all care providers
- Right to have advance directives honored
- Right to designate support persons or visitors
- Right to be free from unnecessary restraints
- Right to participate in discharge planning
- Right to receive written discharge instructions

Patient Safety Protections:

- Right to report safety concerns without retaliation
- Right to receive medication information including purposes and side effects

- Right to infection prevention measures following established guidelines
- Right to continuity of care during transitions
- Right to translation/interpretation services when needed for safe care

4. Insurance and Financial Rights

ACA Protections:

- Right to coverage despite preexisting conditions
- Right to preventive services without cost sharing
- Protection against lifetime or annual limits for essential benefits
- Right to coverage for adult children up to age 26 on parent's plans
- Right to summary of benefits in standardized, understandable format

Claims and Appeals Rights:

- Right to clear explanation of claim denials
- Right to internal appeal of coverage denials
- Right to external review by independent organization
- Specific timeframes for appeal decisions
- Right to coverage during urgent care appeals

Surprise Billing Protections:

- Protection against out-of-network balance billing in emergencies
- Protection against surprise bills from out-of-network providers at in network facilities
- Right to advance notice and consent for out-of-network care

- Right to good faith estimates for self pay services
- Dispute resolution process for excessive charges

5. Complaint and Enforcement Mechanisms

Regulatory Oversight:

- Office for Civil Rights (OCR) for HIPAA violations
- Centers for Medicare and Medicaid Services (CMS) for Medicare/Medicaid issues
- State health departments for facility licensing compliance
- State medical and dental boards for provider conduct issues
- State insurance departments for coverage and claim issues

Complaint Filing Procedures:

- Healthcare facility patient advocate or grievance process
- Provider organization complaint procedures
- Insurance company appeals processes
- Regulatory agency formal complaint submission
- Legal action when appropriate for serious violations

Documentation Recommendations:

- Maintain detailed records of all concerning incidents
- Document names, dates, times, and specific events
- Record conversations and save written communications
- Obtain relevant policies or regulations that apply
- Collect supporting evidence from medical records or witnesses

About the Author

Dr. Bryan Laskin has spent over two decades at the intersection of healthcare, technology, and patient advocacy. As a practicing dentist, he witnessed firsthand the artificial barriers separating dental and medical care despite their profound connections. As a healthcare technology entrepreneur, he's developed innovative solutions to improve care coordination, enhance patient communication, and increase healthcare transparency.

Frustrated by seeing patients struggle to navigate fragmented healthcare systems, Dr. Laskin co-founded Cair, a platform designed to empower patients with control over their dental health information. This technology enables patients to break down the artificial dental-medical divide that compromises comprehensive care.

Dr. Laskin has lectured internationally on healthcare innovation, published two best selling novels, as well as numerous articles on practice transformation, and consulted with healthcare organizations on patient centered care delivery. His unique perspective spanning clinical practice, technological innovation, and system design provides the foundation for the strategies presented in this book.

Beyond his professional credentials, Dr. Laskin brings the personal passion of someone who has navigated healthcare both as a provider and as a patient. This dual perspective informs his belief that healthcare works best when patients are empowered partners rather than passive recipients, a philosophy that animates every page of *Unfair Care*.

Dr. Laskin lives in Minneapolis with his wife and two children, and continues to advocate for healthcare transformation through writing, speaking, Standard development, and entrepreneurship.

Acknowledgements

This book exists because countless patients shared their healthcare struggles and triumphs with me over years of clinical practice. Their experiences revealed both the system's failures and the powerful potential of patient empowerment. To every patient who trusted me with your care over the years, as well as your stories, I sincerely thank you for an education no school could provide.

Special gratitude goes to the healthcare innovators working to transform disjointed care into cohesive healing. Your willingness to challenge entrenched practices despite institutional resistance creates hope for meaningful change.

I'm deeply indebted to my colleagues who bring Cair and our affiliated applications to life, who also reviewed manuscript sections, providing invaluable clinical and systemic perspectives:

Aleh Matus

Megan Hennen

Abby Frey

Nate Johnson

Kseniya Kutukova

Jill Sirko

Dr. Allison Stolz

Most importantly, thank you to Tesa, Naiya and Milcs for supporting this project, along with my many crazy projects, despite the time they demand. Your patience, encouragement, and willingness to hear endless healthcare transformation discussions made this book possible.

Finally, thank you, reader, for your commitment to healthcare empowerment. By implementing these strategies, you not only improve your personal care experience but contribute to the broader transformation healthcare desperately needs. Your refusal to accept substandard care passively represents the most powerful catalyst for system-wide change.

Do You Have a Book in You?

At Glowstick Press, we take your idea from **spark to spotlight**. From manuscript development to design to marketing, we guide you through every step of the publishing process.

We publish and promote books that matter, helping professionals share their insights, stories, and expertise with the audiences who need them most.

If you've ever thought, "I have a book in me," now is the time to bring it to life and make it shine.

Glowstick®
P R E S S

Crack Open. Illuminate.™

shine@glowstickpress.com

www.ingramcontent.com/pod-product-compliance
Lightning Source LLC
Chambersburg PA
CBHW031143020426
42333CB00013B/492